1994

New Dynamics

for

HOSPITAL BOARDS

New Dynamics

for

HOSPITAL BOARDS

EVERETT A. JOHNSON
and
RICHARD L. JOHNSON

Health Administration Press
Ann Arbor, Michigan   1994

Note from the publisher concerning copyright and use of materials contained in this book: We wish to make clear that we reserve copyright on all materials contained in this book. However, we do hereby grant and encourage adoption of the appendix questionnaires within your health care institution and additionally grant permission for the limited copying needed for that purpose, provided that such copies are not for sale or distribution beyond your institution.

98 97 96 95 94   5 4 3 2 1

Library of Congress Cataloging-in-Publication Data

Johnson, Everett A.
  New dynamics for hospital boards / Everett A. Johnson, Richard L. Johnson.
       p.   cm.
  Includes bibliographical references and index.
  ISBN 0-910701-97-0 (softbound)
  1. Hospital trustees. 2. Hospitals—Administration. I. Johnson, Richard L. (Richard Lee), date. II. Title.
RA971.J544   1994   362.1'1'0684—dc20   93-48565 CIP

The paper used in this publication meets the minimum requirements of American National Standard for Information Sciences—Permanence of Paper for Printed Library Materials, ANSI Z39.48-1984.

Health Administration Press
A division of the Foundation of the
  American College of Healthcare Executives
1021 East Huron Street
Ann Arbor, Michigan 48104-9990
(313) 764-1380

Contents

Foreword

In this book, Everett and Richard Johnson take a serious look at one of the most important issues in health administration today: how governance is linked to the critical arena of public policy. With major reforms under way, and more reforms anticipated as the health care debate continues, the timing of this book could not be more appropriate. The Johnsons have always been able to articulate their views to the delight and benefit of many in the health care field, and this work is no exception.

At this historic point in the evolution of our nation's health care system, it is clear that we have reaffirmed health care as a community affair. One outcome of this community focus is that we are placing a stronger emphasis on the process of hospital governance and giving more responsibility to the community leaders who make up the thousands of hospital boards in the United States. Coping with this change and developing policies to guide hospitals through it will require increasing amounts of time and understanding on the part of trustees. The complicated and risky environment of public policy adds a new dimension to the trustee's role.

The Johnsons provide a thoughtful mix of history, current status, and prognosis for health care delivery. Their book includes a proposal for a revised national health policy and much advice on the role, structure, and evaluation of governing boards.

Hospital CEOs will want to share this book with their governing boards and leaders of their medical staffs. The knowledge gained from this book will enliven debates, discussions, and educational sessions in hospitals and health care organizations. Readers will be pleased that they took the time to become acquainted with this latest Johnson brothers' contribution to the health care literature.

Stuart A. Wesbury, Jr., Ph.D., FACHE
Senior Vice President
Tribrook, Inc.
Westmont, Illinois

Preface

Over the past few years, there has been a growing anxiety about where the health care field is headed during the last decade of the twentieth century. When we first entered the health care field, just after World War II, everything was expanding. New hospitals were springing up, older hospitals were adding wings, the future was one of expansion and growth. This sense of a bright future has been replaced with uncertainty about the future of health care and a series of difficult questions that need to be faced:

- If all the abuses in health care are eliminated, will costs continue to rise?
- How much money is really needed to provide health care at an acceptable level?
- Can unnecessary, cumbersome, and inappropriate legislation be repealed?
- What happens to health care economics if everyone is entitled to accessibility and affordability?
- Can hospital governance cope with the coming changes in public policy?

These are the pivotal questions that remain unanswered and therefore lead governing boards of hospitals to have serious doubts about the future when addressing local problems of capital expenditures and uncompensated care. Like it or not, governing board members find themselves having to make assumptions about the direction of public policy when they make long-term decisions affecting their institutions. Although government is a silent partner at monthly board meetings, its influence pervades all major decisions. It is therefore imperative that governing boards have a sense about where public policies in health care are headed.

In addition to knowing about public policy issues, governing boards need repeatedly to examine their own role and effectiveness as an important component of the hospital. Too many hospitals, both public and nonprofit institutions, have remained locked in their traditional organizational structures with rigid positions or mind sets about their role and the responsibilities in governance. Given the rapidity of change in the health care environment, the imperative for board effectiveness lies in knowing the interrelationship between public policy and governance.

For governance it means answering some tough questions:

- Is the governing board too large (or too small) for effective interaction with the chief executive?
- To what extent should knowledgeable health care executives be added to the board?
- Since physicians are periodically recredentialed by the hospital and employees have annual performance evaluations, should board members' individual performances be evaluated annually?

Seeking answers to these questions is difficult. How much money is apt to be needed, how it should be spent, and who should pay the bill is an elusive equation. There is a plethora of opinions but a surprising lack of information on projected health care costs.

Who should be on the hospital governing board, what expectations there should be about performance, and what role the governing board should play are equally elusive.

The conclusions lead to identifying pitfalls to be avoided in proposing solutions for governance and public policy. Hospital governance needs to take a strong stand, based on knowledge and commitment, toward those who propose sweeping reforms in health care. All-encompassing, elegant solutions to problems now facing the health care field will probably be inappropriate and wrong. It would be tragic to watch the best health care system in the world falter and fail because public policies are adopted that cannot be economically sustained. Governing boards can play a major role in assuring that does not happen, provided they recognize what they must do to bring about greater effectiveness. We hope that this book will provide a meaningful basis for helping to bring about sound health care policies supported by local hospital governing boards.

This book is devoted to the intertwining of public policies and governing board issues. This interrelatedness must be understood if the voluntary health care system is to survive.

Purpose

One of the major issues publicly discussed is, Where is health care headed? Other questions are, Will the health care system be nationalized? or Is the Canadian health care system a model for the United States? Every time the news media reports a new solution to the health care crisis, the level of public discomfort with the existing health care system increases. Current health care practices evolved out of an affluent society, but our society is no longer affluent.

There is an urgent need to understand how much money will, in fact, be needed by the health care system in the years ahead. Many of the proposals, such as the Report of the National Leadership Commission on Health Care, focus on the issues of "access to health care for all Americans, cost control, and quality of care," and attempt to develop a funding solution.[1] The Pepper Commission Report on Comprehensive Health Care proposed to "reform the nation's existing system for insuring medical or health care, and [create] a system for insuring assistance in the tasks of daily living that we call long-term care."[2] On 26 September 1990, Representative Henry Waxman introduced Resolution 375 embodying these principles for a national health care plan developed by the American Public Health Association. The resolution included universal access, comprehensive benefits, ability to pay, and cost containment, among other items.[3]

In the same issue of the *New England Journal of Medicine* that reported on the findings of the Pepper Commission, its editor, Dr. Arnold S. Relman, asked the question, "Would the program outlined [in the Pepper Report] really be able to contain the health cost spiral?"[4] He concluded that no one could say for sure, but he believed that only this sort of comprehensive effort has any chance of being successful.

None of the proposals answer the question, Where is health care headed? It seems logical to look at the public policy issues and relate them to the problem of governing our hospitals. The insights obtained could then be helpful in deciding realistic and unrealistic roles for government, insurance carriers, and the providers of health care services. The analysis is revealing.

The overall conclusion moves in a different direction from most of the proposals now being discussed. An elegant, all-encompassing public policy for health care leads away from, not toward, a sustainable public policy in the years ahead. The ability to sustain a health care program depends on financial feasibility. If a universal health care program is desired, then the future costs of this kind of a health care system must be appreciated. When these economics are examined, the results strongly suggest that equal access and equal health care for all citizens is an admirable but unattainable goal. To legislate such a program, relying on federal control and funding, will put in place a system that will be short lived. If such a program is put in place, hospital governance will have to cope with the decisions arrived at, well-meaning but shortsighted.

Efficient hospitals do not just happen, and effective medical care is not a happenstance. The bedrock of strong hospitals and excellence in medical care is determined by capable governance. When a board of trustees knows where it is going and how to get there, competent patient care at a reasonable price is the result.

The problem is twofold: to understand the economics that surround the hospital and how they may affect its role in society and to have in place a governance structure that is capable of guiding our institutions through the treacherous waters that lie ahead in this decade.

Public Policy and Hospital Governance

The modern-day health care system is gigantic in both breadth and depth. To develop an understanding of how it operates and is constrained by public policy is a full-time effort. Too often, myths obscure the realities of its operation. In both public and private sectors, what one believes as fact, whether reality or myth, determines how one thinks about and what one proposes as solutions to the health care crisis. Too often, public policy focuses on a particular provider of health care services or a segment of the health care continuum, rather than understanding that it is an articulated process and interrelated to other parts of the process.

Until the 1940s, hospital boards of trustees had unlimited freedom to establish policies and direct institutions as they chose. Hospitals were unlicensed, malpractice judgments were unenforceable, and physicians were restrained only by their conscience.

Then the Hill-Burton program was enacted and required hospital licensure, the Joint Commission on the Accreditation of Hospitals mandated clinical privileges, and the courts upset the eleemosynary exemption for malpractice judgments. Next, the Medicare program was passed, followed by a steady flow of federal laws and regulations that increasingly strait jacketed past policy freedoms of governance.

The economics of health care are now the drivers for change in the boardroom. Tough decisions are ahead for governance. Given the history of trustee performance, a long, hard look at how governance is functioning is needed.

That requires an assessment of the effectiveness of governance, not just once but regularly, to evaluate corporate and individual board member performance. Competent medical care at an affordable cost is too important to ignore an examination of governance policy and performance.

Hospitals are now moving in directions and at a rate of change never anticipated in the past. Trustee policies and procedures need rethinking for hospitals to provide the scope and depth of medical care now needed. In the following chapters, current problems and future practices are identified and explored. There are no formulas to secure a hospital's future. An awareness of and sensitivity to change and new government mandates, coupled with a depth of health care knowledge, objective analysis, and national decision making, are the best preparations for an unknown future. This book addresses the need to establish a corporate governance culture to avoid simplistic, emotional policy decisions. Hospitals must accept and abide by governmental laws and regulations but center their decision making on keeping patients the center of their concern. And when public policy abuses patients, board members must become spokespersons for patients.

Notes

1. National Leadership Commission on Health Care, *For The Health Of A Nation*, (Ann Arbor, MI: Health Administration Press, 1989), xii.
2. Special Report, "The Pepper Commission Report on Comprehensive Health Care," *New England Journal of Medicine* 323, no. 14 (1990): 1005–7.
3. "The Nation's Health," *Official Newspaper of the American Public Health Association*, October 1990.
4. *New England Journal of Medicine* 323, no. 14 (1990).

Part **I**

Responding to the
Health Care Environment

Chapter **1**

The Health Care Revolution

External factors are now the major change agents in the health care field. Previously, new medical knowledge and technology generated change. For the foreseeable future, the delivery of health care services will be affected mostly by how these services are financed. Physicians, the central decision makers during most of the twentieth century, are being replaced by business and government, who are deciding how to spend health care dollars. During the past decade, the hospital marketplace has become competitive, overbedded, underfinanced, specialized, advertised, market driven, overdoctored, and expensive. Traditional hospitals are in difficult times.

As government and business firms determine how to spend their health care dollars, hospitals have become concerned with the impact of competitor hospitals and other medical care providers in their market area. Physicians were also concerned but still hold, by and large, to their traditional ways of doing business. Price competition and marketing strategies have not yet found their way into the daily language of physicians.

What Is Missing?

Missing is the answer to how much medical care is needed and who will receive the care. Until now, health care providers have remained accountable for medical outcomes, while third party payers and government, who have mandated payment restraints, have ignored the financial well-being of the providers of care. Hospitals have fiercely competed for paying patients. They have minimized services to indigent patients because they cannot afford the accompanying losses.

In the drive to create a price-sensitive, competitive marketplace for health care services, large block purchasers of care are substantially affecting who delivers care, who provides indigent care, and how much can be charged. Third party decision makers have been concerned only with their own constituencies. Lacking a social commitment, third party payers have squeezed out of the medical care system those who cannot pay.

At the same time, the need for cost containment in the delivery of health care services cannot be ignored. An accommodation needs to be reached between reasonable and necessary health care services and the costs for providing them. An equitable way must be found to provide health care for the indigent. A case in point are acquired immunodeficiency syndrome (AIDS) patients.

Block purchasers of health care cannot be expected to be concerned with the health care of those who are not enrolled in their programs. Hospitals, however, make the nightly news when they try to protect their financial position by limiting indigent care.

Historically, hospitals have cooperated with neighboring hospitals, sharing equipment, information, medical staffs, and personnel—just about everything but money. These experiences are now past history. Hospitals have come to understand that conflict is a fundamental element of competition—competition for resources and patients. And competition does not have a zero-sum outcome—there are winners and losers. Hospitals are going through a transition to a market economy while most physicians are still thinking about how things may eventually change.

Typical Governing Board Policies

Four unwritten policies of the past have been upended as hospital executives and boards of directors have tried to cope with a new era:

1. *A hospital was expected to treat competitors, physicians, and everyone else fairly.* Fairness is a feature of an environment of plenty. Competition has caused changes that have significantly reduced a commitment to fairness. Loss leaders are steadily increasing in hospitals, thanks to Medicare and managed care. Sooner or later, and probably sooner, individuals living in smaller communities are going to holler about how unfair it is to have to travel two hours to deliver a baby because their hospital closed.

2. *A hospital provided acute care at one site; all other types of medical care services in the local market were reserved for the entrepreneurs of the medical staff.* Internal warfare may be the order of the day between hospital executives and medical staffs whenever off-site health care ventures, such as an ambulatory program that can be run without backup support services of a hospital, are proposed. Freestanding imaging and diagnostic centers run by hospital-based physicians are now found in some communities across the street from the hospital.

3. *Hospital management kept medical staff problems away from the agenda of the board of directors.* The weakest leadership group in a hospital is typically its board of directors. Whenever there is a medical staff controversy, hospital executives know that the directors will be uneasy about what to do and will frequently support the medical staff, believing they are customers of the institution and therefore cannot be disciplined.

4. *Keep physicians happy and hospitals in the black.* This unwritten policy has been around for the last 30 years. From the 1950s through the 1970s, it was a breeze to meet this criteria. When a problem arose, enough money was thrown at it to keep all interested groups satisfied. As the profligate times disappeared, hard choices needed to be made, and management staffs lost their job security. The situation is now similar to firing the manager of the baseball team because the power hitter in the lineup is in a prolonged slump.

Overturning these four informal policies has made life difficult for both the physicians and management. Executives have accepted the new reality, but clinicians still cling to the past.

Cost-Shifting Effects

Restricted financial diets for hospitals, through the use of preferred provider organizations (PPOs), health maintenance organizations (HMOs), managed care, per capita payments, and discounts, have substantially decreased cost-shifting practices. As opportunities to shift costs fade, the difficulty of providing indigent medical care increases. As business, third party payers, and the federal government struggle to pay only the medical costs of their beneficiaries, provider funding for indigent care decreases.

The Robin Hood theory, practiced by hospitals to compensate for inadequate public funding for the needy, is eventually going to backfire on patients, government, and insurance carriers, but the reaction of each major interest group will be different.

Patients will be affected two ways: quality of care and access. Until a few years ago, the medical profession publicly pushed the notion that, by and large, all physicians were equally competent, as were hospitals. Thinking people knew better. The one serious control on physicians' and hospitals' behavior was malpractice suits. That is not to say that medicine was unconcerned, only that the internal mechanisms were inappropriate for identifying and controlling practitioners of inadequate care. This is still the situation in spite of all the interest in quality of care.

As financial restraints continue to increase, internal controls for maintaining high-quality care will be further compromised. In most hospitals, 20 percent of the medical staff admit 80 percent of the patients. As hospital revenues sink to break-even or loss levels, hospitals will be less and less willing to discipline or discharge a poor quality physician who is a major admitter. In addition, acquisition of new technology is apt to significantly decline. In both instances, quality care will be reduced, to the detriment of patients. Corner cutting may become a way of life in some hospitals facing severe financial pressures.

Patients' access to medical care will be increasingly restricted with the growth in managed care enrollments. As managed care grows, political heat on government will grow as the states and the federal government look for ways to reduce their own health care commitments. State governments will attempt to shift their Medicaid burdens elsewhere, to the federal level or to hospitals. At the same time, the federal government will seek to ease its burden by reducing benefits or increasing fees.

Expected Federal Outcomes

With large federal budget deficits continuing for the foreseeable future, Congress will look for ways to dump their problem on business rather than on private citizens without resorting to a national health insurance program. Congress appears to have learned the lesson that when health care is established as a political right, the control of health care expenditures is lost. The Medicare program is a lesson in point. Congressional representatives are well aware that a vote either to reduce coverage, to increase individual payments, or to install a means test will meet with considerable resistance from the affected electorate.

A social program that exceeds the public's willingness to accept new taxes, pay higher premiums, or accept larger deductibles or coinsurance forces deficit financing and only increases the federal deficit. Recognizing this reality means that the responsibility for funding health care benefits is apt to fall on insurance carriers. Even though the states regulate insurance carriers, the federal government is adept at finding ways to override state regulations.

A likely result is that the federal government will establish a national standard for private health insurance policies. The following could be included in the requirements:

- Provisions for greater access for needy, part-time employed, handicapped, and high-risk patients
- Uniformity of minimum health insurance benefits
- Protection from catastrophic illness expenses
- Portability of benefits
- Community rating versus experience rating

Should these be required as federal mandated policies, health insurance carriers would face a new set of difficulties. Implementing such requirements would be up to the insurance industry. That would permit Congress to avoid the line of political fire.

The time for major health care financing changes appears to be drawing closer. Health insurance premiums continue to increase rapidly. The expense control strategies of the last 15 years—deductibles, coinsurance, experience rating, PPOs, HMOs, utilization reviews, managed care, and DRGs—have used up their savings potential so that provider cost increases once again become straight passthroughs to the policy holder and health care expenditures keep growing as a percentage of the gross domestic product (GDP).

With existing cost control strategies no longer able to slow down cost increases, a reordering of hospital and physician relationships is the place to look for future cost reductions. Other than the closed-panel HMOs adopting different arrangements, insurance carriers have only gingerly explored new possibilities.

From the viewpoint of health insurance, it makes sense to aim toward having one provider payment for both hospital and medical services for an episode of illness. In the past, the medical profession has quickly sunk this idea. The latest try at integrating hospital and physician payments was a trial balloon floated by Medicare.

Various types of package payments will increasingly be explored. The amount of change will be directly related to the severity of the economic threat. There are growing signs that accommodations can be made with physicians.

Medical Staff Issues

The inability of hospital executives to deal effectively with physicians arises from the historical development of an organized medical staff in the hospital. The medical staff concept became widely adopted in 1919. In 1897, only 2 percent of the physicians had hospital privileges, and most physicians practiced medicine as a secondary endeavor to a primary income, such as farming. As basic medical knowledge of anesthesia, asepsis, and surgery developed, medical practice provided sufficient income to become a full-time career.

The American College of Surgeons provided leadership to improve care in hospitals and established the Hospital Standardization Program in 1919. In 1951, this accreditation program was transferred to the Joint Commission on the Accreditation of Hospitals (now JCAHO).

Because the Hospital Standardization Program required physicians to form an organized medical staff, hospitals asked for a model set of medical staff bylaws. By 1950, it was rare to find a hospital that had not adopted these model bylaws word for word, and the idea of an organized medical staff was imbedded in hospitals.

These bylaws structured the medical staff as a self-governing body with a separate line of authority to the governing board. The organizational result of this long chain of events is that, even today, the chief executive of a hospital has no formal authority over the medical staff component of the hospital. This organizational structure has become more awkward and unworkable as external pressures increase on hospitals. Governing boards' unwillingness to deal with medical staff issues of quality of care, appropriateness of care, or physician fees erodes the usefulness of the present organizational structure.

The health care field is undergoing major shifts in financing, public attitudes, the availability of nurses, surpluses of selected specialties of physicians, and technology improvements that are moving patients out of the hospital to ambulatory care programs. Yet the hospital organizational structure remains locked into the form of the past.

As hospital resources are strained, conflicts with medical staff increase as physicians join to form special interest groups pressing demands for their own specialties. Institutional survival depends on resisting unreasonable demands.

The traditional separation of hospitals and physicians presents difficulties in the negotiation of a preferred provider arrangement with an insurance carrier. Physicians, particularly hospital-based physicians in cardiology, radiology, anesthesia, and pathology, may refuse to sign a participating physician contract. Often, their hospital contracts do not require them to participate as part of the hospital contract with the insurance carrier, so they remain separate and bill at their regular fees rather than at the discounted rate in the contract.

As the present trend intensifies, situations will arise in which insurance carriers and hospitals work together to overcome medical staff resistance. When a large number of patients are available under an insurance contract, closer hospital-physician relationships like the following will be encouraged:

- Large, multispecialty medical groups entering into exclusive contracts with hospitals
- Single-specialty group practices entering into exclusive contracts for total coverage of that specialty in hospitals
- Capitation payments made to specialty groups through a hospital for a managed care contract

These concepts may be unthinkable today for most hospitals and physicians, but as health care finances steadily become more restricted, the unthinkable will be considered. Economic well-being is a great motivator.

When a hospital governing board is faced with a large loss of revenue because a physician group decides to move its hospital practice elsewhere, a board may well accept a third party carrier's proposal to grant an exclusive arrangement. A sufficient patient volume and commensurate revenue to replace what is being lost is an attractive alternative.

The rationale for physicians turns on a different issue since they are aware that the traditional freedoms of the medical professions are being eroded. Clinically, they are experiencing limitations in medical care judgments as managed care, PPOs, and utilization reviews have expanded. In addition, professional charges are now subject to fee screens, discounted fees, the loss of referral freedoms, and relative value payment systems.

Physicians recognize that when both medical judgments and fees are restricted, professional freedoms are reduced. They sense that these control mechanisms are likely to be transitions toward even more onerous controls. These controls are a source of frustration since most physicians chose a profession rather than a business career, but they now find that the controls force them to behave as if they were small business enterprises. Along with their interests in the medical profession, they are also concerned about their own personal welfare. When physicians are financially secure, they can express a greater concern for the profession than for their personal lives.

However, younger physicians are open to nontraditional methods and ways of working with insurance carriers and hospitals since they have not been hardened by past experience and relationships.

In the past few years, a new marketing strategy has appeared that is likely to grow and change the organization of medical practice. Brand name medical practice has expanded beyond home base. The Mayo Clinic now has operations in Jacksonville, Florida, and Scottsdale, Arizona, while the Cleveland Clinic has an outpost in Fort Lauderdale, Florida.

Public response to brand name medicine has been enthusiastic because these familiar names stand for high quality medical care in people's minds. Because of this reputation, schedules in the new locations have quickly filled. In addition, if you are a Mayo or Cleveland Clinic patient, you receive only two bills: one from the hospital and the other from the clinic for professional services. Patients appreciate not receiving the customary five or six individual physician bills for professional services, particularly when they may never have seen some of the physicians from whom they received a bill. As brand name medical practices prosper, it is probable that existing groups with 30 or more physicians are likely to follow the Mayo and Cleveland Clinics' example and open subgroups in adjacent areas. In those cities with brand name clinics, local hospitals and their medical staffs are busy at improving service and quality, yet they are competitively handicapped because their physicians are independent practitioners and have no mechanism for consolidating professional fees into one bill.

The next few years are going to see additional difficulties and conflicts. If hospitals and physicians can successfully provide medical care at an affordable price, the credit will probably be due to insurance carriers actively reorganizing existing health care relationships. If hospitals and medical staffs continue to struggle over financial turf, the resolution of issues will be slow and lag considerably behind public expectation. Since insurance carriers control a large proportion of the funding for health care, their active interest will speed up the required realignment of interests.

Chapter 2

Twelve Lessons from Corporate Restructuring

When economic competition between hospitals began to flourish, freestanding community hospitals rushed to convert to parent-subsidiary-model structures. This organizational form enabled hospitals to operate both for-profit and not-for-profit activities on multiple sites under one control. The initial wave of conversions has now passed; in its wake remains the question whether corporate reorganization has been a sound course of action. Some who made the transition would do it again; others would not. Still others have reversed these decisions and collapsed multiple organization structures into a single hospital corporation. In short, corporate restructuring has encountered growing pains; some were inevitable while others could have been avoided. When the health care organizational landscape is surveyed, there are 12 major lessons to be learned about corporate restructuring.

What Is Corporate Restructuring?

In its simplest terms, corporate reorganization is a realignment of resources (human, material, and financial) to enhance competitive strength. The two most common types of reorganization for a freestanding hospital are to either vertical or horizontal structures. In a horizontal reorganization, the traditional hierarchy is repositioned to a new set with equal partners in a relationship at the top of the organization. In health care, a common example is to place the community hospital on a horizontal line with several other hospitals, with all institutions operated as subsidiaries of a parent corporation. Investor-owned chains of hospitals (e.g., Hospital Corporation of America) have followed this pattern. A horizontal organization provides similar services at multiple locations to capture differentiated market segments over a geographically widespread area.

The other common strategy is vertical integration. This organization focuses on developing and controlling a comprehensive range of health care services, ranging in intensity from critical care to subacute care, to provide a full spectrum of health care services in a community. This continuum may be loosely connected through a system of collegial referrals or tightly managed with detailed determinations on the use of resources.

Over time, vertical integration is usually enhanced by additional marketing strategies to protect the system from competitive threats. In addition, improved system economies of scale are developed by activities such as a purchasing program for expensive, highly specialized technical diagnostic units for computerized axial tomography (CAT) scanners, lithotripters, or radioisotope drugs that may be incorporated within existing organizational structures or as new entities depending on anticipated volumes. Strategies to capture market segments often include setting up a captive insurance carrier or an HMO to reach specific pools of patients. Real estate corporations may be added to develop further links with medical staff members, through medical office buildings and ambulatory care facilities.

Whichever reorganization strategy is commenced and whatever form it eventually takes, the reason for system reorganization remains unchanged: to provide a structural hierarchy through which strategic market niches are acquired and resources are economically deployed throughout the system.[1] In the wake of health care reorganizations, however, a variety of conflicts have emerged over the past several years to impede strategic success. Twelve sources of conflict have been identified:

Lesson #1: Reorganization should be based on anticipated market and environmental conditions—not fad or fantasy.

An organization not faced with threats to survival or recognizable opportunities for growth may not need to reorganize. Alfred Chandler demonstrated 25 years ago that organizations move through a sequence of developmental phases when responding to changing market conditions.[2] When an organization is not required to respond to a market or the marketplace does not change, a static structure often suffices. Examples are public bureaucracies that are guaranteed survival by law. In other situations, when the community hospital is the sole provider of hospital care and is protected from competitive threats, the traditional organizational structure continues to serve them well. In most circumstances, however, that is no longer true. A fundamental issue, then, is determining when reorganization is appropriate.

Critical to effective restructuring is an objective, valid, and timely assessment of the real-world environment. All too often, hospital or medical staff leadership will deny the existence of market threats. Sooner or later, the hospital leadership finds itself vulnerable to competitive forces that have been developing over several years. Declines in occupancy may be wrongly attributed to a national trend when, in reality, a nearby hospital is increasing market share at the expense of one's own hospital. Changing medical technologies that are improvements over existing technology offer opportunities to capture new markets (particularly outpatient markets) to organizations who get there first.

A combination of market opportunities and threats typically motivate reorganization. If no opportunities exist, the organization is likely to prefer the status quo; if no real market threats are imminent, there is little motivation for organizational change.[3] Without external stimuli, the process atrophies.

Conclusion #1

It is usually too late to commence reorganization efforts after the competition has gained significant market strength. Market assessments need to be conducted in advance of significant competition because the costs of transition are turmoil and fragility. Boards must act with foresight and courage in assessing a need for reorganization. Strategic market forecasts, comparative analysis of competitive behavior, regional health care trends, and emerging technological opportunities should be the measures of organizational performance used to indicate the value of reorganization.

Lesson #2: Form follows function.

A key reality in the reorganization of a hospital is that structure is always a dependent variable: form follows function. New or revised structures alone do not create anything; neither do new market shares, new economies of scale, or new loyalty from patients, physicians, or providers. The success of reorganization is uniquely dependent on the competitive environment in which a hospital or health care system functions. Restructuring must be developed according to a strategically relevant environment, an often debatable subject. For example, a hospital board may argue that their relevant environment is the primary service area from which the hospital draws its patients. The medical staff may argue the environment consists of several geographical areas depending on the reputation of various clinical programs. The hospital chief executive may define the boundary based on competitor analyses and expansion opportunities for new programs and services.

Conclusion #2

Developing a shared commitment among major participants in the hospital is critical to the assessment and implementation of reorganization. Commitment to the health care mission and strategic service boundaries is developed over time by mutual participation and success. Annual retreats for the board, the medical staff, and senior management help prepare for strategic decision making in the face of competition. Meetings, more meetings, and still more meetings are required to ensure all the major participants remain committed through the difficult planning and start-up phases.

Lesson #3: For effective reorganization, the interdependency of corporate units must be clearly acknowledged.

Having a valid, future-oriented strategic analysis and commitment to a clearly agreed on service area is not sufficient for reorganization. The need for restructuring usually occurs when the hospital's primary patient service base erodes. Hospital chief executives have recognized that the traditional response to offset a decreasing hospital occupancy level is to expand the comprehensiveness of services. In the past, when specialized departments were developed to meet patient needs, traditional departmentalization along functional lines was adequate. Hospital executives now know this approach no longer fills hospital beds. Motivated by an erosion of the traditional patient care base, hospitals have attempted to capture more patients from larger geographical areas. In pursuing this avenue, an inherent inefficiency arises: indirect and fixed costs of providing services through the creation of several subsidiary corporations drains revenue sources. Even after systems are reorganized, this dilemma often continues when the cash-cow hospital has its revenues diverted to units that operate unprofitably. Recognition that the survival of the hospital depends on the development of local or regional systems is an important precursor to reorganization.

Key leaders in decision-making roles are subject to a second pressure. Hospitals have traditionally been organized along dual lines; hospital departments and clinical departments of the medical staff are parallel structures that do not provide for integrated decision making. The resistance to coordinating clinical and administrative information has created a highly inefficient decision-making structure. In all but the most serious patient care matters, the medical staff committee structure still attempts to maintain the medical staff as an entity independent from the rest of the hospital. New mechanisms for interdependent strategies and operational decision making are now required. Reorganization may be used to separate clinical decisions from business decisions. The hospital can focus on quality of care issues while the parent corporation concerns itself with the economics of the system.

A third pressure for reorganization comes from a hospital's need for additional sources of revenue and multidisciplinary problem solving. Medical staff members often simply do not believe hospital resources are limited; they may argue that the cause is poor management or a proliferation of unneeded management services. In days past, when hospital resources were ample, it was easy to develop more and more decentralized hospital departments, a typical growth pattern for the last 40 years in U.S. hospitals. Limited resources coupled with competition have forced a search for new alternatives. Limited resources demand economies of scale that can only be realized through collaborative, integrated plans. In the absence of economic pressures, physicians vigorously resist efforts to restrain their independence. In the past, patients, physicians, and hospitals did not need to monitor costs seriously under the cost-reimbursed payment system. Resources are currently being deployed along product lines, increasing the difficulty of using traditional department-based budgets.

Conclusion #3

Before undertaking corporate reorganization, the presence of three criteria for successful reorganization should be assessed: (1) a critical demand for specialized services over a wide geographic area; (2) a need for rapid, interdependent decision making in complex tasks; and (3) competitive pressures for economies of scale with flexible, shared use of human resources.[4] If these conditions do not exist, reorganization will probably not work better than traditional organizational arrangements.

Lesson #4: Reorganization efforts are much more costly and politically charged than they appear at first.

When restructuring became popular in the health care field, the major rationale used to persuade governing boards to authorize multiple corporations was to circumvent certificate-of-need regulations. As patient days began to decline across the nation, resulting in lower occupancy rates in hospitals, another major concern rapidly surfaced: a desire to develop additional sources of revenue by establishing both nonprofit and for-profit subsidiaries. In the course of planning an organizational shift from a one-hospital corporation to a health care parent-subsidiary corporation, a latent motivation for reorganization emerged. It often occurred to hospital chief executives that reorganization provided a way to reduce the size of the large, constituent-representative governing boards to whom they reported. Since large boards often necessitate chief executives spending between 25 and 50 percent of their time on governance matters, the possibility of creating a smaller strategic board of directors through restructuring had considerable appeal.

Once key decision makers were sold on approving a new corporate structure, the problem of developing a consensus among board members became important. When considering how the board members were likely to vote, reorganization advocates tended to focus exclusively on securing the needed votes. Attention to three essential and controversial factors was often overlooked or minimized: (1) the reserved rights of the parent corporation, (2) the size of the parent board, and (3) the board's composition. The emphasis on securing votes obscured the need for a full exploration of how these three factors would affect corporate organizational effectiveness. The unspoken principle was that whatever was undetermined at this first stage of board and corporate transition could be corrected later, when the major organizational building blocks were in place.

The result of this superficial, often politicized development process was a series of vague assumptions about board responsibilities and interrelationships. As a result, the reserved rights of the parent body were often minimized. It was often assumed they would not be implemented. To ensure the desired result of maintaining hospital dominance, the size and composition of the parent board often included all members of the hospital board, whose inclusion contributed to role conflicts and ambiguity in the new structure.

Conclusion #4

Reorganization is a means to an end with long-term potential for market strength. The inherent political costs must be considered side by side with the potential gains in competitive strength. Without a significant opportunity for success in the marketplace, the political upheaval in the transition phase will likely reverse reorganization initiatives.

Lesson #5: Reserved rights must be clearly defined if reorganization is to be effectively implemented.

Experience has indicated that the reserved rights of a board need to be clearly delineated and accepted before a transition takes place to prevent false assumptions being made about how the new organizational structure will operate. The delineation of reserved rights should spell out the following:

- The purpose and goals of the multicorporate structure
- The control of the articles of incorporation and by-laws of each subsidiary corporation
- The creation of additional subsidiaries, mergers between subsidiaries, and the dissolution of subsidiaries
- Defined dollar amounts permitted subsidiaries for asset purchases, sales, leases, and mortgages
- The approval of the selection and the removal of directors of subsidiary corporations
- The selection of legal counsel and an auditing firm
- The development of a strategic plan for the corporation
- The approval of business plans of subsidiaries
- The approval of operating and capital budgets of subsidiaries
- The determination of the uses of surplus funds generated by subsidiaries

The delineation of the reserved rights of a parent corporation presents no difficulty in the creation of subsidiary corporations but is a major hurdle with respect to the hospital. In moving to a parent-subsidiary model, an existing hospital corporation must vote itself out of being a corporate entity (exercising the full range of rights) into a subsidiary that has limited authority. This is doubly difficult because the hospital must finance the operations of the new parent corporation and provide working capital for any additional subsidiaries. In the formative years, when additional monies are needed and the use of the excess funds generated by the hospital are determined by the parent board, hospital board members often resent being the cash cow. This resentment is compounded when hospital board members perceive that they lose some authority when the parent-subsidiary relationship is formed. Conversely, when reserved rights are spelled out, a hospital board may remain the primary decision-making body for controlling the assets and surplus funds that are the only viable sources of support for the parent.

Conclusion #5

All concerned must accept the reserved rights of the parent if the parent-subsidiary model is to be effective.

Lesson #6: The purpose and composition of the parent governing board must be distinguished from subsidiary boards.

Because of the sensitivity that surrounds the issue of the reserved rights of the parent corporation, some organizations have elected to have all the hospital board members as board members of the parent corporation. A variation of this approach is where members of the executive committee of the hospital are named directors of the parent corporation.

The rationale for this duplication is twofold. First, since hospital funds are the main source of financing subsidiaries, the hospital board maintains control to ensure these activities support rather than conflict with those the hospital undertakes. Second, the hospital governing board wants to ensure the hospital activities remain the major concern of the restructured corporation.

Behind these reasons there is an underlying attitude of hospital board members. If they are expected to agree to the restructuring and also put up the money, they are going to control how the money is spent. In reality, this kind of thinking makes the parent corporation a subsidiary of the hospital and effectively defeats the purpose of creating the parent-subsidiary organizational model.

Confusion exists in the minds of many board members, who then perceive that the two boards are doing exactly what they did when they were only one board. It often takes a year or more for the majority of board members to have this perception. Their conclusion is that the only accomplishment has been the creation of unnecessary duplication. Usually, a board is slow to form this opinion. At the time of transition, the key group guiding the restructuring assures all concerned it will take some time before the boards develop a smooth working relationship, so skeptical board members wait for all the good things forecast to actually occur. When they do not within a reasonable period of time, the skeptics tend to vocalize their feelings and concerns. Doubt and anxiety may come to dominate an already fragile situation. Persons selected for the parent board and the hospital board should differ in their characteristics. Parent board members should be analytical, objective, and broadly knowledgeable about the health care field. Hospital board members may typically be more operationally oriented, with a hands-on approach to their responsibilities.

150,386

Conclusion #6

Parent governing boards should devote their efforts to long-range planning, coordination, and finance, while subsidiary boards should concentrate on operational and quality of care issues.[5] Parent and subsidiary board members require differentiated roles and requirements. Parent board members must be competent at a systems level in thinking and planning, in large-scale corporate strategy, and in policy development. Subsidiary board members need to have expertise in operational matters such as quality of care, finance, community relations, and corporate leadership.

Lesson #7: Clarification of roles and relationships between the parent and subsidiaries is critical.

In a parent-subsidiary model, the parent is a nonoperational entity. Even when the parent corporation's reserved rights and authority to determine the use of funds are understood, the acceptance of the hospital governing board's limitations of authority often remains a problem. This is a serious difficulty that emerges from a nonprofit organizational philosophy. Nonprofit hospital boards have traditionally been representative of their communities, and board members have considered it their primary responsibility to measure all of their decisions by the yardstick of community interests. Because they are unpaid, they see themselves as providing voluntary community service and are often unwilling to acknowledge a higher authority exists in the parent-subsidiary corporate setting. The new organizational structure takes away their decision-making authority for determining community interests and leaves them in the role of only making recommendations on operational matters. Hospital board members do not usually foresee the loss of this right when they vote to adopt the parent-subsidiary model.

By the time it becomes obvious to members of both boards that the organizational structure is not working properly, a year or more has passed. Those who orchestrated the transition will come to appreciate the difficulty of modifying a structure that is flawed because concessions were made or neglected while they were trying to secure enough votes to establish the new model. An attempt to remove substantial overlap and ambiguity in membership roles is needed when the hospital has 90 percent or more of the total assets and provides all the working capital. A dilemma arises when business judgment conflicts with emotional attachments to the traditional ways of decision making at the hospital board level. Once organizational structures are codified in bylaws, they are almost impossible to change unless situations develop that threaten the existence of the corporation. Short of that point, bylaws are cast in concrete.

The parent corporation's role is strategic, concerned far more with what is ahead than with what is happening today. It uses past results to correct the course of the future by allocating resources to bring about the desired end results. To a great extent, the parent board is a think tank that explores and evaluates ideas. It requires participants who are widely experienced and have considerable breadth in the health care field. Their talents need to be mixed with those who have demonstrated entrepreneurial skills, business acumen, and community acceptance. As a body, the parent board needs to be composed of compatible members who enjoy the concentrated thinking required to formulate and analyze proposals and who have experience in strategic negotiations among powerful interest groups. Far from being ritualistic and formal, the meetings of this body need to be freewheeling, all-day affairs, usually quarterly.

Conclusion #7

Recognize that clarification in the distinct roles of the parent board and the hospital board is not accomplished by just explaining differences. Clearly defined concepts evolve out of carefully developed agendas that lead board members to accept their changed roles and, in turn, support the strategic plan, as well as to accept the reserved rights of the parent.

Lesson #8: Confront unrealistic expectations of success through up-front planning, negotiation, and creative problem-solving.

When a parent-subsidiary model is adopted, an aura of relief and optimism may prevail. There are expectations of plenty of health-related business opportunities just waiting to be recognized, acquired, and moved into the appropriate slots on the organizational chart. The anticipated result is a synergistic effect among all of the related health companies rapidly leading to substantial profits. Disappointment usually sets in after a year or two when the cumulative results are studied and show expenditures have been substantially in excess of revenues. Then the question what happened needs to be addressed. False assumptions, primarily related to a lack of planning, were made and believed.

Conclusion #8

Realistic business plans need to be prepared annually for each subsidiary and reviewed quarterly.

Lesson #9: False assumptions about corporate staffing needs create internal system warfare.

In some cases, the chief executive of a hospital becomes the full-time chief executive of the parent corporation, and the former chief operating officer takes over as chief executive of the hospital. Whether or not the chief executive position of the parent is a full-time position often lacks careful evaluation. The assumption is made that once the position is created, it becomes a full-time position. However, the result may be unexpected problems. Even though the parent staff may consist of only the CEO and a secretary, the immediately incurred expense is substantial. If subsidiaries other than the hospital exist, they are usually in the formative stages. Identifying new opportunities, buying related companies, starting companies, employing personnel, and generating new revenues all take more time and money than originally estimated. By the end of the first year, the operating costs are often far in excess of the revenues from these new activities.

The expense problem is compounded when several persons are added in this formative period, such as a chief financial officer, a director of marketing, a director of planning, and necessary support staff at the parent level.

In addition to the salary costs, a decision may be made to house the parent staff at an outside location, necessitating the leasing of space and the purchase of furniture and equipment. This further widens the gap between expense and income. A corporate staff is typically appointed from the ranks of current hospital managers. While familiar with the health care field, they may lack experience in building businesses or in evaluating existing businesses for possible purchase. This lack of experience often leads to overly optimistic marketing projections. In turn, optimistic forecasts lead to paying higher purchase prices for related activities. Reflection might lead to a decision to call a halt and retrench.

A second source of role conflict soon emerges when corporate staff are employed in a parent-subsidiary model. Personnel at the subsidiary level might perceive a duplication of executive functions. This perception is particularly nettlesome in the executive ranks.

Experienced, long-term executives in flagship sub-sidiaries see the parent executives as interfering with sub-sidiary turf, a source of considerable friction. When the flagship subsidiary is also funding corporate staffs, the du-plication of roles adds insult to injury.

Conclusion #9

Realistic evaluation of corporate staffing needs and re-sources must be considered in the context of parent-subsid-iary impact on existing human resources. One alternative may be to have hospital executives assume shared respon-sibilities at both hospital and corporate levels until the cor-porate positions evolve into full-time jobs.

Lesson #10: Don't underestimate the need for physician support.

In general, physicians do not favor the transition to a par-ent-subsidiary model. They correctly interpret this struc-tural change as putting management one organizational step further away from the medical staff. This interpreta-tion is projected into an assumption that executives will be less likely to be influenced by physicians' interests and opinions. The feeling of distance is increased when senior management moves out of the hospital and off the premises to another location.

Health care corporations that have adopted the parent-subsidiary model have, for the most part, ignored or denied the attitudes of physicians on this subject. Unlike hospital matters, where there is usually a higher degree of consider-ation for physicians' viewpoints due to clinical issues, par-ent governing boards have often adopted the position that the structural transition was made for business and eco-nomic reasons. They then attempt to assure physicians that they should not be concerned unless they can demonstrate, in some tangible manner, there has been an adverse impact on patient care. Such patronizing exclusion merely unlocks latent distrust among the medical staff.

Conclusion #10

Physicians correctly view themselves as crucial to the success of the hospital and, in turn, to the success of the parent corporation. Significant interest and time should be spent to secure and maintain physician support for a successful transition to a parent-subsidiary organizational structure. The role of the physician on the hospital board is to provide significant insight into quality-of-care issues. At the parent board level, the role of the physician is more ambiguous. From the standpoint of the medical staff, the physician board member is the guardian of their interests and important to securing continued medical staff support for the restructured corporation.

Lesson #11: Management skills and understanding developed solely out of a hospital background may be inadequate for personnel decisions in subsidiaries.

As the parent health care corporation adds for-profit and not-for-profit subsidiaries, the chief executive is forced to wrestle with a new set of problems. Having spent many years in the not-for-profit hospital, the parent chief executive has grown accustomed to the existing salary scales and fringe benefit patterns of the hospital industry. When subsidiaries are added that are heavily marketing-oriented and for-profit driven, prevailing income patterns may be commissions or salary plus bonus. This difference poses an adjustment problem for the executives who must approve salary schedules. They are predisposed to continue the patterns with which they are most familiar.

The adjustment becomes more difficult when the new positions must be staffed by personnel—such as sales representatives, stock brokers, or freelancers—from industries where conditions and incomes considerably vary with hospital standards. When these new positions typically have higher incomes and do not require graduate degrees, the temptation has been to employ young, minimally experienced persons from other industries to protect the salary and fringe benefit structure of the hospital. The results obtained are what would be expected—less than desirable. Learning curve problems are encountered that would have been avoided if more experienced persons had been employed. Unfortunately, a year or two passes before such judgments can be made. The inadequacy of the results is often due in large measure to inexperienced managers being placed in charge of these subsidiaries.

Conclusion #11

Do not insist on salary scales and fringe benefit patterns being tied to hospital standards. Instead, use income and benefit patterns appropriate to the activity.

Lesson #12: Competitive strategies must be analytically determined and must not be token efforts.

Having lived most of their professional lives in a cost-reimbursement climate, many chief executives of not-for-profit hospitals have had false notions of economic competition. When diagnosis-related groups (DRGs) were adopted and a fixed price per hospitalization begun for Medicare patients, many hospital chief executives feared the worst. However, their initial fears were not realized. Instead of hospitals immediately suffering reduced revenues, they began experiencing the largest surpluses ever in the history of hospitals. This led many hospital chief executives to view economic competition with enthusiasm and delight and re-inforced their desires to be economically competitive. Some regarded the new environment as a game in which it would be easy to be successful. Having encountered no difficulties in the early stages of economic competition, it was viewed as an easy avenue. Additional successes could be obtained by developing health-related subsidiaries such as nursing homes, retirement centers, freestanding surgical centers, primary care centers, or physicians' practices. Because a subsidiary's economic failure had little financial impact on the parent or hospital corporation, the unspoken strategy was to beat the neighborhood hospitals in the game of friendly competition. It became more important to win an acquisition than to be strategically directed toward fulfill-ing the mission of the corporation.

The excitement of the game sometimes became para-mount; maintaining parity with competing hospitals be-came the prime motivator. Rather than treat potential ac-quisitions as straightforward economic decisions, all sorts of rationales came into vogue to justify these pursuits, including

- purchasing physician practices in the service area to maintain market share;
- guaranteeing income levels to specialists needed to round out the complement of specialists on the staff;
- buying smaller, outlying hospitals to use as a refer-ral network for tertiary care;
- expanding the modalities of care to include home health care and hospices;
- providing sports medicine services;
- developing wellness programs; and
- selling durable medical equipment.

The intention behind all these efforts was to make a practicing physician more interdependent with his or her hospital, thereby protecting its market and revenue generating ability. Even when pro formas showed questionable profits or indefinite unprofitability, efforts would be undertaken if there was the slightest possibility of an increase in patient days. As a result, a consolidated parent-subsidiary profit and loss statement often showed the hospital turning a substantial profit. Meanwhile, all the other subsidiaries showed losses, even before allocations for indirect expenses were calculated.

These results were discouraging but should have been expected. The euphoria of trying something new—moving from benign cooperation to frantic competition—blurred the risks inherent in new ventures. Instead of carefully nurturing one or two ideas to maturity, there was a rush to put the corporate structure into place and then look around for appropriate opportunities. At the strategic level, it was a classic example of form before function. When anticipated results were not quickly forthcoming, frustration emerged and was gradually replaced with a realistic, discouraging lesson in understanding the grim cycle of economic competition.

As yet, most of these reorganization attempts and unsuccessful ventures have not fatally wounded hospitals. The flow of operational revenues from patient services has not yet seriously declined. But as Medicare funding reacts negatively to inflation and the Health Care Financing Administration (HCFA) further restricts hospital payments, the resulting financial pinch will require the reevaluation of each subsidiary. Those in the red will be discontinued or sold at nominal prices. If enough are not breaking even, the question of returning to a hospital corporation as the sole enterprise will resurface and be reexamined.

Conclusion #12

Before commencing a subsidiary, determine its financial feasibility and the period of time required to break even.

Employ a chief executive officer (CEO) for the subsidiary with the understanding that if the timeframes, budgeted revenues, and expense are not met, the subsidiary will be discontinued.

Outcomes of Reorganization

The process and outcomes of reorganization in health care are exceptionally complex and difficult to achieve. A hospital board or executive that attempts to illustrate that the future survival of the hospital depends on integration of any sort, whether it be internal or system reorganization, is met with denial. Success in such efforts heavily depends on the amount of environmental pressure, the perceived need for interdependent decision making, and a desire to share limited resources from a multidisciplinary perspective. Some health care systems have moved in this direction, although the struggle has been hard. Forces that make reorganization appropriate from a strategic level are often removed in both time and impact on day-to-day operations. It is extremely difficult to secure medical staff support because it is an arena in which they have little familiarity. An all-too-frequent reaction to reorganization is to kill the messenger by terminating the chief executive or recalling the board. Such actions are only an effort to deny the need for change and realistic adjustments.

Finally, after chief executives have experienced the parent-subsidiary corporate model and its challenges, it is unlikely, in the event of failure, they will lead their organizations back to providing inpatient care at one location. Having developed a frame of reference around multiple health care activities on multiple sites, these executives are going to continue to think in the same terms. They have experienced new dimensions in health care and find such experiences to be personally satisfying. Health care corporations are likely to remain on the scene, but their growth may be slower than was anticipated a few years ago.

A few will revert to their original hospital corporate structure or will be absorbed into local or regional health care corporations. Most of those who have adopted the new corporate model will stay with it, dropping those subsidiaries that are money losers and being more cautious about commencing new ventures. They will pay much more attention to up-front strategic planning. Once a business plan is begun, greater time and attention will be devoted to ensuring its projections.

Thus, in spite of the corporate restructuring experience to date, continuing competitive forces and hard-won executive experience have propelled us beyond the single corporate hospital structures of yesterday. Complex health care systems will continue to emerge regionally and locally. But going back again is impossible; strategic wisdom must replace romantic notions of quick success in a competitive marketplace.

With the formation of local health care systems and new strategies to tie physicians more closely to one system, subsidiary joint ventures were developed between the hospital and physicians of the medical staff. These joint business ventures subsequently raised ethical questions in Congress and elsewhere. If the new multifaceted health care corporate systems are to reach their ultimate potential, the ethical considerations of economic relationships between hospitals and physicians must be faced.

Notes

1. J. C. Goldsmith, *Can Hospitals Survive? The New Competitive Healthcare Market* (Homewood, IL: Dow Jones-Irwin, 1981).
2. A. Chandler, *Strategy and Structure: Chapters in the History of the Industrial Enterprise* (Cambridge, MA: MIT Press, 1962).
3. A. L. Delbecq and P. Mills, "Managerial Practices That Enhance Innovation," *Organizational Dynamics* 14, no. 1 (Summer 1985): 24–34.

4. S. M. Davis and P. R. Lawrence, *Matrix* (Menlo Park, CA: Addison-Wesley Publishing Co., Inc., 1977).

5. S. L. Gill and A. L. Delbecq, "Developing Strategic Direction for Governing Boards," *Hospital & Health Services Administration* 33, no. 1 (Spring 1988): 25–36.

Part **II**

Redefining Leadership
Roles and Relationships

Chapter 3

Restructuring Hospital Governance

With the costs of hospital services projected to increase steadily and federal fiscal policy to become more conservative, hospital governance policy decisions will become more complex. Now that hospitals have multicorporate structures, the chaining of operations, off-site businesses, and discounting rates to a variety of third parties, past organizational accountabilities and authorities will no longer be appropriate.

Since governance and chief executives are on the cutting edge of these adjustments, they must find new opportunities. Should they fail to adjust, the organization will not cope well with new circumstances.

Up to the present time, there are no published studies that report in detail the total number of hospitals in the country reordering their governance functions and those of the CEO. However, through our daily interactions with a wide variety of hospitals, it appears that the majority of institutions are doggedly holding on to yesterday and making only piecemeal adjustments when faced with a crisis. The proof of the pudding is the current number of hospitals in poor financial condition.

In many situations, the CEO was aware of the likely future outcomes but lacked the courage to force change or was stymied by a governing board that was unwilling to face community and medical staff pressures. Only a relatively small number of hospitals have been able to cope successfully with the risks that are a part of the process of change. Indeed, it does not seem likely that the percentage of risk-taking organizations will increase. Ten years from today, the future institutional survivors will be those hospitals' organizations that have revised their top organizational structure through a systematic and thoughtful process, based on a willingness to compete in a new market environment.

Changes in the Nature of Responsibilities

How will responsibilities shift? Whether or not a hospital chooses a multicorporate structure or elects to remain a single corporate entity, the role and nature of the functions of the governing board and the CEO must be different than those traditionally practiced, if they are to survive.

A governing board's composition and function must be altered for a successful future. How these adjustments will be accomplished is less important than the end result of reordering the functions and judgments of the board of directors. By nature, voluntary nonprofit hospital trustees are conservative and reluctant to give a higher priority to business rather than social policy, yet the imperatives of current market changes require a shifting of priorities. However, the unique characteristics and values of quality medical care must continue to be recognized no matter which orientation is primary, if the public is to continue to value hospital care.

The traditional hospital governing board has a mixture of experience, perspective, and skills. Policy decisions are too frequently delayed or permanently deferred because a significant number of directors, generally with diverse motives, cannot reach a unified position. When this situation arises, no action is often the result.

The essence of a useful policy body for a hospital is a governing board composed of persons who are capable of coping with complex issues, think objectively, and understand the milieu of medical care. In a boardroom, the primary criteria for deciding a policy matter should be the good of the hospital, not how it affects an individual director or his or her friends. Too often, quality patient care and sound financial decisions lose out to parochial interests. A "play it safe" approach to policymaking is usually the end result of the traditional stewardship philosophy that permeates the orientation of typical hospital directors and blocks reasonable risk taking for new market opportunities.

In a period of rapid change in organizational functions and rising competition, a standpat perspective frequently has greater long-run risks than a willingness to be venturesome. A successful risk taker is one who more accurately assesses the probabilities of success and failure than a competitor. Sensible risk taking is hard work if one is to recognize the controlling issues, evaluate their impact, and develop workable strategies and tactics.

New Criteria for Board Selection

The historical criteria for selecting hospital directors have been what community group a person represents, what specialized experience the person possesses (e.g., lawyers, bankers, business leaders), whether the person is a woman or of a particular religious persuasion, or whether the person is influential in the medical field. None of these criteria are hinged on a quality of mind that has been deepened and broadened by wide experiences in our society.

There typically is a naive expectation that a diversity of community interests among directors will become of secondary importance when hospital affairs are considered. The reality of a boardroom is that specific areas of interest are of greater importance to directors than the well-being of a hospital.

As the intensity of competition increases in the future, a hospital will need to become more selective in assessing the personal abilities and characteristics of its board members. The quality of mind and the composition of a successful hospital board of trustees in the future will be significantly different than those of present day boards. Future boards will have the following characteristics.

Limited board size

The exact number of members is less important than the criteria that the size of the board be sufficiently small to allow time for each director to express opinions on each agenda item. When the criteria for selection is on the quality of intellect and an ability to understand complex issues and to think objectively, an opportunity to express individual opinions becomes critical.

The inclusion of top executives

The CEO, chief financial officer, director of patient services, chief operating officer, and perhaps the director of marketing may be gradually added to the board of directors as the complexities of operations, financing, and off-campus businesses become increasingly important to a hospital.

Permanent medical staff chiefs

With the growth in managed care, PPOs, and independent practice association (IPA) HMOs, the wisdom of establishing permanent chiefs of service will become obvious, even to those physicians who have believed that rotating chiefs were their best insurance for maintaining the freedom of private practice. The impact of discounting fees will sooner or later force them to protect their remaining practice by joint hospital and medical staff bidding on discounted fees and rates.

Rotating medical staff leadership

The board of directors will probably continue to provide ex officio membership to the president and the president-elect of the medical staff as a way to appease the residual fee-for-service physicians. If they lack an ability to think broadly about the hospital's evolving role, that will gradually work to reduce the other directors' esteem of their value to policymaking decisions, so that their impact on policy decisions will steadily decrease.

Outside members

Voluntary hospital boards will have a difficult adjustment to the idea that trusteeship is no longer the essence of stewardship. However, as market opportunities are lost and financial difficulties increase, there will be an increasing awareness that survival requires greater understanding and abilities than can be expected from the historical source of leadership.

The future trend will be to consolidate the internal leadership of the hospital as part of the board of directors with selection based on their positions in the hospital organization structure. This change will require that major clinical chiefs be appointed by the governing board for relatively long tenure periods, rather than be based on annual elections by the clinical departments of the medical staff.

The chairperson of the board may or may not be the CEO. On some voluntary hospital boards, the tradition of community leadership will prevail as a residual of the stewardship concept. In other instances, where there has been rapid growth in both size and complexity, the CEO may become chairman of the board as a full-time position.

The Changing Committee Structure of the Board

To accommodate the need for additional input sources, the committee structure of the governing board will have committee members who may not be board members. The chairperson of each committee will be appointed from the membership of the governing board.

The committees of the board will be limited in number to the following standing committees: the executive committee, the finance committee, the nominating committee, the marketing and planning committee, and the professional relations committee. The use of five standing committees is based on the need to have greater depth of knowledge and expertise in these areas than can be expected from the wide scope of responsibilities assigned to the governing board; therefore, additional nondirectors' skills can be focused in specific areas.

With a small number of directors, it is possible to avoid establishing an organized committee structure. However, it is also a political reality that a governing board needs to assure that the hospital's constituencies understand, accept, and support its decisions. Involvement in preliminary discussions and input into decisions generally are useful ways to ensure support.

Committees will function within broad areas of delegated authority so that a governing board can primarily operate to coordinate and evaluate hospital functions. This delegation will require substantial changes in the board's usual agenda. More emphasis will be on informational items—new technology, market opportunities, capital acquisition, quality control, and competition. There will be an increase in reports summarizing and evaluating operations. Procedural items will be consolidated to save time.

Committee reports will not be debated in detail, as is customary in traditional board meetings, but quickly evaluated for their fit into the overall strategy of the hospital and adjustments made when necessary.

The number of meetings for both the board and its committees will be more limited than in the past. With broader administrative authority, the need for frequent meetings decreases, but each meeting will be longer in length as the board concentrates on future plans.

In multicorporate hospitals, subsidiary boards of directors will be composed primarily of members of the administrative staff. They will function as divisional operations of the parent with coordination and control centered in the office of the CEO.

In essence, the governance structure of successful hospitals in the future may closely resemble a typical corporate board of directors of successful business firms.

The Role of the Chief Executive Officers

As the role and nature of governance changes, so will the characteristics, functions, and skills of a hospital CEO.

The control of the medical staff

Probably the greatest change that will occur in this position will be a growing degree of authority in directing the administration of the medical staff. The growth of PPOs and IPA-type HMOs, plus the wide-spread adoption of DRG-type reimbursement and a variety of hospital-physician joint ventures, will create a need for greater centralization of decision making. Physicians will maintain clinical freedoms in the practice of medicine, but economic imperatives for discounts, utilization controls, and integrated health care businesses will drive the administrative aspects of medical practice into a closer relationship with the CEO.

Because a governing board needs to formulate rapid responses to market opportunities, it will be required to delegate a greater degree of authority to CEOs. This delegation will avoid the typical time delays caused by routing decision making through a standing committee to an executive committee and finally to the governing board.

An increase in the number of operating factors to consider will also broaden the CEO's area of executive decision making. Because of an increasing complexity of interrelationships between operating issues in an environment that is unpredictable, more hands-on control will be required.

Board members should no longer view the title of president as an ego builder for the CEO but as a reflection of the reality of changed conditions. Vice-presidential positions are expanding for the same reasons. A president does not have the depth of knowledge required to direct the internal functions of the major divisions of the hospital and its related businesses. The result is a greater delegation of authority. Good judgment is the hallmark of excellence.

Future sources of chief executive officers

Like in other types of endeavors, the route to the CEO position will be less predictable. Master's programs in health administration will continue to provide candidates for the role of president but will not be the only route. Future presidents will require at least two types of knowledge and skill: the education provided in master's of business administration (MBA) programs as well as the industry-specific knowledge acquired in a health care management curriculum.

Candidates will also require greater strength in at least one major functional area: marketing, finance, or operations. There will be a decreasing emphasis on the clinical knowledge a physician possesses. The emerging model of a president requires an understanding of the traditional value systems of health care and knowledge of how good medical care is evaluated. The expectation that this knowledge can be acquired only through a medical education and experience will gradually diminish at the top level of management.

Market strategies and negotiating skill will become recognized as necessary attributes of a president. The role of the senior executive staff will be as sources of expertise needed to frame the parameters of what is achievable within the limits of financial feasibility.

As more and more hospitals go from $50 million to $200 million a year enterprises, governing boards will increasingly seek replacement executives among members of the existing staff. The cost of a poor selection will be increasingly apparent because of the involvement of senior executives on the governing board. Their skills will already be known. When an incumbent president fails to adequately plan for succession, hospitals will resort to a greater use of executive search firms to find a replacement.

Conclusion

The days ahead will be much different than the past. How well a hospital survives and performs in the future will, in large measure, depend on the acceptance of change in the structure of governance and executives.

The two questionnaires in the appendix to this book can be used to survey the governing members of your hospital and to gather their input on ways to improve leadership. The surveys might also be useful as educational tools for physicians, board members, and executives.

As external forces create the need for modifications in the traditional role and function of the governing board, new stress will be placed on the relationship of the chairperson of the board to the CEO. Board members do not now recognize many of the nuances of this relationship. Because future organizational change depends on an understanding of the chairperson-CEO relationship, the typical characteristics and effects of this relationship need to be considered.

Chapter 4

The Relationship of the Chairperson of the Board and the Chief Executive

The relationship between the chairperson of the board of a hospital and the chief executive is rarely discussed. Common sense precludes a CEO from publicly expressing opinions that may later be heard or read about in a hospital's local community. Yet the consequences of the interrelationship of these positions is important to the success of a hospital and to the career of a CEO. In nonprofit hospitals, a public member of the board of directors is typically the chairperson, elected for a specified term of office, while a career professional is the CEO for an indefinite period based on performance. Investor-owned hospitals usually combine both positions in one individual and are not concerned with this relationship, but one should remember these hospitals constitute only 10 percent of the total of the nongovernmental hospitals.

Changing Authority and Responsibility

With the shift to economic competition between hospitals, managed care, and discounting, there is an urgent need to realign the traditional formal and informal organizational relationships between the chairperson of the board and the chief executive.

In many nonprofit hospitals, the activities of individual directors and chairperson may create major operational difficulties for CEOs. In some hospitals, the governing board may be too deeply involved in management affairs and make decisions on matters without adequate insight and knowledge of how these decisions affect operations. When this happens, unnecessary problems are created for the CEO, who must then proceed to develop workable modifications and spend considerable time in this effort. In essence, concerned amateurs are forcing a CEO to spend unnecessary hours of effort to accommodate a less than well thought out decision. This effort creates excessive time demands on a CEO and takes away from time that could be spent on hospital operations.

In some hospitals, decisions of the governing board put the CEO in the position of having to exceed delegated authority to cope with an immediate problem. Since a board meeting is informally controlled by social niceties, the limits of the CEO's position are typically not a matter for debate in front of the full board.

Since the operational climate of a governing board is not rigorously established and controlled, a new chairperson usually does not have a strong sense of the specific limits of the office. In addition, there is a desire to create one's own position and image. Many chairpersons are at, or near, the top of a business firm, and they tend to operate as a line executive rather than as a chairperson. This behavior preempts a CEO's position.

Because a chairperson is aware and is often reminded by physicians that a medical staff is self-governing, there is a temptation to deal directly with the medical staff. Since members of the medical staff are appointed by the governing board, they may bypass the CEO and bring their concerns directly to the chairperson. This bypass is risky since an inexperienced chairperson may compromise hospital policies and strategies without meaning to do so.

The heart of the matter when a chairperson deals directly with a medical staff is a lack of knowledge about medical affairs and practices. A chairperson may not know what he or she does not know and therefore willingly accept the viewpoint of physicians as representative of the best interests of a hospital.

An experienced chairperson who accepts the limits of the office and adheres to the duties as defined in the bylaws does not strain relationships with the CEO. When the chairperson's authority and responsibility are not clearly defined, the potential for misunderstandings is always present.

The chairperson of the board is the first among equals as presiding officer of the board of directors. Under parliamentary procedure, the chairperson votes to break tie votes of the board, an exceedingly rare occurrence.

Typical position responsibilities for a chairperson as defined in hospital bylaws are

- providing leadership to the board to ensure that the activities of the board and committees are within the authority granted by the articles of incorporation, the bylaws, and adopted policies;
- approving agendas for and scheduling board meetings;
- inviting board members and arranging through the CEO for hospital executives or outside experts to provide information and opinions related to the board's area of deliberation;
- ensuring that deliberations of the board are directed toward recommending policy and not toward making operational decisions; and
- appointing directors to participate on standing and special committees.

Typically, bylaws enumerate no specific authority and responsibilities for the chairperson but define accountability to be to the board of directors. The chairperson's term of office is usually limited to one to three years with tenure either limited or unlimited. In most instances, the bylaws state no qualifications for the chairperson.

Less Than an Equal

Conversely, the duties, authority, responsibility, accountability, qualifications, and tenure for a chief executive are specifically stated either by bylaws or a position description. Even though the CEO may be a voting member of the board of directors, other directors usually perceive this position as less than an equal position, since the CEO is the agent of the board.

The same perception also affects the chairperson-CEO relationship, both consciously and subconsciously, because the CEO seeks advice and support from the chairperson. Both perceive the essence of their relationship as a delegation of authority from a superior to a subordinate. While a chairperson frequently seeks advice and support from the CEO, implicit in the relationship is an awareness that whenever the chairperson indicates a course of action, it is an order, even when given with grace and charm. Conversely, when the CEO suggests a policy direction, the chairperson is not required to accept this suggestion. The fact is that their relationship is often one way. If a CEO wins support at a board meeting over the objection of a chairperson, there are two major risks: a loss of respect from other directors for poor manners in taking a strong stand or the possibility of antagonizing the chairperson with potential long-term consequences for the CEO. If the issue is a fundamental one, a CEO's win may cause the chairperson to resign, while a CEO's loss may result in a termination.

A typical hospital directors meeting is often controlled by carefully observed social protocols that constrain even mild disagreements as a breech of acceptable social conduct. Where such practices exist, a CEO is required to state a position delicately and to avoid highlighting a significant difference of opinion with a chairperson. Unless a CEO can privately persuade a chairperson to change an opinion, there is no other forum for a thorough review of facts to objectively arrive at an optimal decision. Occasionally, another director can be quietly encouraged to take up the CEO's position and influence a chairperson to change an opinion. However, the formal organization mechanisms of a governing board are not structured to handle diversity. Back channels encourage the use of informal, invisible ways of seeking compromise.

The Need for Continuity

A successful hospital requires stability and continuity in its leadership positions. Since nonprofit hospitals typically rotate the chairperson of the board position among directors every few years, the CEO is expected to provide long-term leadership. A chairperson usually has a primary business interest elsewhere and has limited time for hospital affairs, while a CEO is full-time and intimately involved in daily hospital activities. To a degree, this expertise strengthens a CEO but can be used on policy matters only within the limits established by the chairperson.

For pragmatic reasons, a chairperson usually delegates authority for executive decisions to a CEO without attention to the authorities and responsibilities enumerated in the bylaws. The functions a chairperson delegates to a CEO are typically informal and evolving. Because chairpersons change every few years, the authority and responsibility delegated to a CEO changes with each new chairperson. These shifts go unrecognized by other directors.

Because the chairperson-CEO relationship is generally friendly and informal, the decision elements of problem identification, defining alternatives, and control elements are almost always unrestricted for the CEO. Frequently, the implementation of a decision remains with a CEO, although the timing of execution might remain in the control of the chairperson or restrictions might be placed on execution. A typical restriction is not to implement a decision until some other action or decision has occurred.

The most frequent decision element a chairperson controls is the selection of a particular alternative, which may be either to do nothing or to select a specific option. A decision by the chairperson not to act often prevents referral to a committee.

Usually, all major hospital functions are delegated to the CEO with two exceptions: financial functions may be limited for nonbudgeted items (by a dollar ceiling) and for changes in senior executive salaries. With regard to medical staff affairs, the CEO is limited to making recommendations to the board and has no authority for implementation. In spite of this limitation, a board of directors may hold the CEO accountable for all the administrative affairs of a medical staff.

Holding a CEO accountable for medical staff matters has been traditional in hospitals since self-governance became common. As long as hospitals had ample resources, this lack of CEO authority was not unworkable, except in cases of egregious physician behavior or a gross lack of control for poor quality medical care by a medical staff.

As hospitals move steadily into an increasingly competitive marketplace, the lack of expanded CEO authority for finances and medical staff affairs is a handicap for the hospital. The rapid pace of change requires timely decisions and rapid commitment of resources by a hospital to enable it to take advantage of new opportunities before competitors enter a perceived new market.

Eliminating Role Ambiguities

In hospitals with a conservative chairperson who believes yesterday's successes will continue in the future and who is more concerned about avoiding risks than succeeding, a progressive CEO will be blocked from capitalizing on new market opportunities before competitors begin operations.

The traditional functions of a chairperson as the presiding officer at board meetings, appointing committees, and overseeing the activities of the CEO is usually obscure and not defined. Consequently, role ambiguities exist for both a chairperson and a CEO.

A chairperson does not know which CEO activities to monitor or the extent to which particular actions should be supervised. On the other hand, a CEO is unclear about the limits of delegated authority and responsibility because restrictions and expansion of both occur piecemeal over time. In addition, a chairperson may informally direct a CEO to deal with medical staff matters or may restrict the CEO's financial decision making.

As the leader of a governing board a chairperson has a duty to maintain and be sensitive to board actions that implicitly modify the established organization structure. When the consideration of an issue implies a change in the authority or responsibility of either the medical staff or the CEO, the chairperson should insist that a realignment of authorities and responsibilities be dealt with as part of the contemplated decision.

It is not a question whether or not organizational adjustments are required but rather an insistence on a clarification of the authority and responsibility of the CEO or of the role of the medical staff. If this type of decision is ignored, particularly when the board directs the CEO to be responsible for a function delegated to the medical staff, the result is a gradual increase in a feeling among physicians that the CEO is usurping their turf and increasing his or her own authority. For example, a board may direct a CEO to limit patient admissions from a physician who routinely exceeds the DRG ceilings. When a board restricts the financial authority of a CEO on a given issue, the management staff is apt to believe that this restriction subsequently applies to all financial matters of a similar nature.

A particularly difficult problem may be created when a chairperson holds a CEO accountable for a medical staff attitude created by a board decision. An example is when a board decides to terminate a hospital-based physician and the medical staff takes up the cause of their colleague. Physicians typically respond by directing their criticism toward the CEO through informal conversations with directors, by portraying the CEO as having engineered the termination. They often buttress this belief by citing poor communications with the medical staff, indicating to board members the CEO is ultimately wanting to take over control of the medical staff. Often a governing board believes such comments and fails to respond by indicating the decision was one the governing board made. In such circumstances, board members may fail to ask for information that substantiates the physician's comments. An inexperienced chairperson is unlikely to be aware of the consequences for the CEO when board members hear such comments. When the chairperson position rotates frequently, a chairperson will probably never acquire sufficient sophistication to avoid these types of organizational traps.

Rotating the Chairperson

A CEO faces a major psychological difficulty every time the chairperson rotates. The CEO must adjust to the personality and ego needs of a new chairperson, learning to adapt to a new set of abilities, strengths, weaknesses, performance, and behavior. A rounding off of sharp edges of the two personalities takes place. This process is usually more difficult for the CEO than the chairperson, because the expected standard is for a CEO to adjust to the chairperson and not for the chairperson to adjust in a major way to a CEO. At the same time, the administrative staff expects the CEO to continue to function as before. That may not be possible if the new chairperson imposes changes that disturb previous management patterns and relationships.

Such changes are particularly difficult in those hospitals where a CEO has delegated to the senior management staff broad areas of authority and responsibility if a new chairperson desires to closely supervise the management decisions. When that occurs, the previous tolerance for error, consensus building, and open communication are replaced with work pressures, conflict, and a restriction of information.

Conclusion

The relationship of a chairperson and the chief executive often has a substantial impact on a hospital organization. When nonprofit hospitals are in a competitive marketplace, this relationship must achieve a higher degree of performance and stability than has been traditionally true.

In this rapidly changing environment, the old standard of keeping the hospital in the black and the physicians happy is no longer the rule of thumb. Today, a CEO cannot maintain these relationships when physician incomes are declining and a hospital is seeking to expand into off-campus health care activities. Unless governing boards are willing to delegate increased authority to CEOs and support them when medical staff pressures arise, hospitals are not going to be able to replace decreasing revenues from inpatient services. Seeking off-campus health-related revenue often affects services typically offered in office practices of physicians on the medical staff.

In the future, governing boards may consider appointing their CEO as chairperson of the board, particularly when hospital finances seriously deteriorate. The day of a part-time chairperson, inexperienced in health care, controlling the decision of a full-time, trained, and experienced CEO and senior management staff is rapidly passing. While concerned citizens will continue to contribute time and talent to a hospital, these factors alone are not adequate for coping with the complexities of a modern-day hospital.

Chapter 5

Mission versus Margin: Religious Hospitals and the Nonprofit Dilemma

In the past decade religious hospitals, of all of the not-for-profit hospitals, have had the most difficulty in dealing with the conflict between their mission and their margin. To protect their net profit has meant paying less attention to the reasons an institution exists as a part of the ministry of healing. The persons on the firing line in a religious hospital are the senior executives who must decide how to balance philosophical ends with income. Hospital positions that only deal with direct patient care are not confronted with this problem, nor are the leaders of the religious order to the same extent as the chief executives of religious hospitals. The continuing pressure under which religious hospitals must function, year in and year out, is unique and needs to be understood at all levels in the hierarchy of the church.

The Good Old Days

Most hospital executives share a desire to return to the good old days when organizational life was less complex and stressful. Personal and community values were consistent with a religious hospital's organizational priorities: expanding access and providing high-quality care to the poor and underserved. Maintaining the church's philosophical objectives posed no difficulties. As the economic climate has changed, organizational priorities have dramatically shifted. Groucho Marx, a sometime American philosopher, aptly described such changes when he said, "It isn't so much that hard times are coming, as it is that soft times are going."

In the days of yesteryear, religious hospitals had governing boards entirely composed of sisters; beds were full most of the year, and hallway beds were a common sight in the winter months. Cost reimbursement programs were the major source of revenue. Indigent care was a minor burden because cost shifting was an honorable activity and physicians were more concerned with patient care than with malpractice. Demand exceeded the availability of beds, and the hospital struggled to take care of an overflowing number of patients.

In the expansionist 1950s and 1960s, health care finances were in good shape. The number of religious members was adequate, and the public appreciated their services. Those times were exciting and rewarding, and the future was rosy. The religious had little difficulty being comfortable with their vows. Both the public community and the religious community were in harmony. The ministry of healing was alive and well. Both religious and organizations were comfortable with their sense of success and satisfaction.

Times Changed

In the 1980s, the age of economic competition arrived, and the traditional fabric of the health care field began to unravel. No longer was it possible to adhere to a single guidepost of serving any and all who needed care. The ministers of healing now had to pay equal attention to the financial aspects of health care. To survive, not only did a hospital have to do good, it had to do well. Financial responsibilities became as critical as social concerns for fulfilling the religious mission. The struggle to do good and to do well came under siege through changes in federal government payment policies for health care. Hospitals were forced to reexamine programs and services and, in the case of religious hospitals, to also reexamine their missions.

New Structures Appear

Three simultaneous and conflicting major forces were affecting religious hospitals: their finances became severely constrained, a need for religious members trained and experienced in governance and management skills grew, and the number of religious vocations declined.

As all hospitals began to face economic competition, critical financial imperatives required organizational changes in traditional hospital structures. The parent-subsidiary corporate model gained favor, as did hospital alliances, to preserve and acquire resources where mission depended on margin.

For years, many religious hospitals had been part of a hospital and health-related system, but most did not have a corporate staff. Business coalitions, Medicare's adoption of DRGs, and a rapid expansion in managed care and other types of competitive medical plans triggered the move to develop corporate staffs with a corresponding multiplication of governing boards. At the same time, religious orders experienced a significant decline in membership. Filling all the newly created governing board seats required a new look at the available number of religious. The growth in board seats exceeded the availability of trained and experienced personnel, which forced a reexamination of governance.

Religious health care was faced with a major challenge to their historical traditions. The societal role of their hospitals had to be balanced with fiscal considerations if these institutions were to survive. The acceptance of both objectives, up and down the organizational chain of command within orders, was difficult. Sisters who managed health care responsibilities for orders were painfully aware of revenue shortfalls and knew health care finances would become even more restricted in future years. These sisters were apprehensive because institutional survival depended on dollars as well as dedication.

Among sisters not directly accountable for operating hospitals, there may exist a feeling that too much emphasis is placed on financing issues to the detriment of social responsibility and the religious mission. In-depth understanding of the complex and ever-changing nature of financing health care is usually only important to the handful of sisters who manage or govern hospitals. Other religious members often do not understand, or choose to disbelieve, the financial and operational realities that come with owning and operating hospitals in the current environment. As a result, a widening schism may develop between religious leaders with hospital management responsibilities and those who do not have day-to-day contact with hospital operations.

Cultural Levels

In many religious orders, there are now four distinct operating levels from which sisters may be drawn for serving on governing boards.

Organization	*Norms and climate*
Sponsoring order or community	Religiously driven
Health care corporation	Market driven

Hospital   Professionally driven
Departmental activity   Operationally driven

In the current environment, these levels have very different cultural norms and climates. These differences are profound and have a lasting impact on those who spend their working years in any one of them. If a sister is a hospital departmental manager and also serves on a governing board, she is most likely to bring her religious and departmental experiences to bear on any issue dealt with by the governing board. In a like manner, a sister serving as a hospital chief executive is apt to act from her over all hospital responsibilities because she has hundreds of employees depending on her management judgments.

When the governing boards of a health care corporation and its subsidiaries are composed of both religious and laypeople, two different cultural climates become mixed. Decisions that start out as market or professionally driven often end up as religiously driven if the matter under consideration is ultimately decided at the top of the corporation.

In religious organizations, it is important for the religious cultural climate to prevail. If, on the other hand, the cultural climate is market driven or professionally driven, a governing board's decisions will, of necessity, reflect this culture.

Balancing Dual Missions

The traditional organizational techniques—clearly defined roles, position descriptions, carefully articulated missions and objectives for each unit and subunit—provide only partial answers for leaders of religious hospitals. For them, the tried and true methods of enhancing decision making are inadequate. Scarce resources require judgment, and judgment comes from organizational experience. Any board member lacking an adequate understanding of the hospital's operating climate needs to be educated, which requires substantial time commitments to be effective. Religious values, by themselves, no longer guarantee the survival of a health care organization.

As hospital revenues become tighter, the religious mission of an order must be balanced against an economically driven marketplace, which often becomes a real source of difficulty. No useful purpose is served by thinking one is more important than the other; both are essential. When financial matters are secondary to religious values, a hospital may fail and jeopardize religious stewardship. While religious values are vital, they must be balanced with a concern for market share, discounting prices, and bonding programs for physicians. If economic concerns become too important, an important social value is lost in the religious hospital. Working for profit is often regarded as unseemly, if not contrary, to service values. Yet sisters in health care executive roles must have a bottom-line orientation, even though other sisters who serve in religious roles may view them as having lost their way.

Professionals in a nonprofit organization often have an inaccurate perception of the business of business. Business leaders are often negatively stereotyped as individuals who are short on honesty and long on a willingness to take advantage of others because they have a flexible set of ethics. Successful business leaders adhere to high ethical standards, even in the most trying of competitive situations. They are acutely aware that value must be added year after year to their products and services. The computer industry demonstrates this point. Hardware and software have become measurably better each year, while consumer prices have been reduced year after year. Customer costs are down and product quality increased with an added value for the consumer as the result.

Surviving economic competition with high ethical standards is a difficult assignment. In today's hospital, the lesson is simple: providing needed community health care services goes hand in hand with good business practices. Because of the changes in the external environment, both the social mission and the financial responsibilities must receive equal attention.

Impact of Cultural Values on Decisions

Four cultural climates affect most decisions that are approved at different levels of governance in religious health care organizations: religiously driven, market driven, professionally driven, and operationally driven. Assume a hospital governing board is considering a $15 million project proposed by the chief executive, a religious, to renovate several nursing units. The proposal is to convert double occupancy rooms to private accommodations to enable the hospital to generate more revenue from patients with commercial insurance, which will affect the number of Medicare and Medicaid patients that can be hospitalized. Through the conversion, the hospital will be able to remain profitable for the next several years. The hospital governing board makes this decision because it is operationally driven. The decision is based on anticipated financial results from attracting patients who can afford to pay or who have commercial insurance for their care.

When a religious hospital is a subsidiary of a local health care corporation, a hospital governing board's recommendation is forwarded to the next higher organizational level for review. At this level the decision will be discussed in terms of market strategy. Board members will want to know if there is a real demand for the recommended types of accommodations. In addition, this board will want to satisfy itself that a $15 million capital expenditure is the best use of dollars from a strategic standpoint when competing with other hospitals in the local area.

Because of the size of the investment, the next level of governance may have to agree to the expenditure. At the level of the sponsor, the proposal may be viewed quite differently. Questions like the following may be raised:

- What will happen to the Medicare and Medicaid patients who will incur more limited admissions?
- Should the alternative of using this money to establish clinics in low income areas of the city be followed?
- Should this money be used to support sponsor-owned failing hospitals operating in the inner city or a rural area?

As the project moves from one governing level to the next, differences in cultural climates become apparent. The questions raised at the sponsor level will lead those at the hospital to believe that financial realities facing the hospital are not understood. At the sponsor's level, there is a different perspective. They wonder why the hospital board has forgotten the mission of the order. Each wonders who's wearing what hat.

Public Perceptions

In addition to different cultural levels, public opinion must be considered, a difficulty confronting all nonprofit community hospitals. If a public poll were taken, it would probably report that religious hospitals and other nonprofit hospitals have a responsibility to take care of all patients who come to their doors whether or not they have the ability to pay. Since hospital charges have risen rapidly over many years, the public tends to believe hospital financial coffers are full. They are often unaware that profit margins have narrowed and are likely to disappear for many hospitals. Nor is the public aware that 44 percent of all patient days are now paid for by Medicare and hospitals are reaching the limits of the revenue shortfalls that can be absorbed.

When religious hospital executives understand the public's attitudes about hospitals, it becomes difficult to budget increased revenues year after year for fear the public will think of the religious hospital as having lost compassion for the poor and needy. Reinforcing the religious mission in the face of declining revenues becomes more difficult each year.

Differing Imperatives

With stiffening economic competition, the imperatives of professional- and market-driven cultures are likely to be increasingly out of step with the religious-driven culture. An unpleasant question arises: To what extent can decisions for a subsidiary hospital unit be made by a parent governing board with a differing cultural climate without risking the effectiveness of the subordinate organization?

The current dilemma facing religious orders that own and operate hospitals is how to continue to meet their religious mission when the environment dictates that institutional survival depends on full-paying patients. This is a single question with two sides: (1) Can governing board members of hospital subsidiaries that must operate in a market-driven or professionally driven environment carry out the religious mission without unduly compromising the mission of the order? and (2) Can subsidiary governing boards effectively respond to the professionally and market-driven climates and still remain true to the mission of the order?

There are no clear-cut answers to these questions. The questions are tough because they require reconciling religious missions and financial imperatives, a complex task that means reframing and redefining long-standing philosophies and traditions. To some, it is unpleasant and distasteful. Others will be frustrated by the uncertainties that must be considered in forecasting the future.

At the same time, the efforts of religious orders must be invested in the future. It is a chance to break with the past, to find innovative and exciting ways to carry out the ministry of healing. The discipline and clarity that come from spiritual inquiry can provide a solid foundation for meeting the challenges of reshaping traditions, hopes, and plans. Such discipline along with grace, gentleness of spirit, and a dedication to a higher calling will enable religious hospitals to meet and surpass their current level of contribution.

Conclusion

New answers and greater heights are the goals for tomorrow and the decades ahead, and achieving them will require an assessment of the performance of the governing boards of religious hospitals. The way governing boards of nonprofit hospitals are structured to meet the economic demands of our times is the topic of Chapter 9. Readers may find that some of the ideas in the chapter can be applied both to religious hospitals and to other types of nonprofit hospitals.

Chapter 6

Ethical Considerations of Economic Relationships between Hospitals and Physicians

When reading a hospital journal, one is likely to find articles describing how to develop a closer relationship between a hospital and physicians that benefits both parties. Toward that end, these articles usually have one or two sentences that say, "by the way, be careful about the ethics involved."

In the past, the tradition and ethics of medical care placed the welfare of patients foremost and the interests of hospitals and physicians as secondary. As long as the financing of medical care was essentially unlimited for both patients and providers, it was easy to maintain an ethical medical standard.

When a major shake-up in Medicare payments occurred in the mid-1980s, both hospitals and physicians began to seek new ways to protect existing revenue levels and to develop new revenue sources. The result has been an expansion of contractual relationships between hospitals and physicians that has focused on economic incentives and bypassed traditional medical ethics.

As competition and regulatory pressures increased, public concerns arose about the ethical behavior of hospitals and physicians toward patients. These concerns center on joint ventures and insurance arrangements.

The public's expectation of ethical behavior in medical care defines the conduct of both the medical profession and the hospital organization and is an expression of the moral standards of society. In the past, physicians and hospitals have publicly professed that the patient's interest was ahead of their own interests.

As the public becomes aware that some hospitals pay physicians for admitting patients to their facility or make nonrepayable loans to physicians, confidence in the integrity of hospitals and physicians has been lessened or lost.[1] The public's reaction to joint ventures of hospitals and physicians for imaging centers, ambulatory surgery facilities, urgent care entities, home health care programs, and home intravenous services is an open question. Large financial returns on limited investments may well erode public confidence in such arrangements.

Numerous examples have been reported of both excessive charges and overutilization of diagnostic laboratories.[2] A 1983 Michigan Blue Cross study reported fees at laboratories owned by referring physicians were almost double the fees of other laboratories.

Less often recognized and discussed, but still open to questions about conflicts of interests, are jointly or separately sponsored HMOs and PPOs with investments by hospitals and physicians. Withholding a percentage of a physician's fee is customary practice for HMOs and PPOs. HMOs and PPOs sponsored by insurance carriers give physicians incentives to take less time with patients and limit diagnostic procedures. The incentives are designed to reduce usage by sharing the savings. There are immediate and powerful incentives to encourage the underutilization of medical care to reduce expenses. In spite of these incentives, both medically sponsored and carrier-sponsored HMOs and PPOs have collapsed because of financial problems. These failures do not reflect weak incentives but the fact that physicians pay more attention to a patient's health than they do to the financial health of the managed care organization.

Physicians are trained to consider all the diagnostic and treatment possibilities for a patient. The economics of medical care become secondary. The fear exists, however, that even though physicians' concerns are primarily clinical, managed care programs may ultimately override physician decisions and compromise patient welfare. The other side of the coin is that fee-for-service medical practice provides strong incentives for treating patients and can lead to the overuse of physician services because of their discretionary judgment in diagnostic and treatment procedures for patients. This is also patient abuse, from the other end of the scale.

Further removed from public awareness is the present practice of hospitals buying physician practices. In 1988, a Hamilton/KSA survey of 600 hospitals reported that 18 percent of hospitals were buying physician practices.[3] When hospitals purchase physician practices, they are interested in increasing or assuring a continuation of patient admissions. This provides incentives for physicians to make admissions that might more appropriately be made to another hospital better equipped to handle a specific type of clinical problem.

Also obscured from public view is the competitive ownership struggle between a hospital and multiphysician groups over new technology, resulting in inefficient duplication of services. The loser in such a contest may be the public because of inequities in applicable regulations that do not require physicians to obtain certificates of need, or to control their utilization and pricing structures.

These new challenges to ethical standards of medical care are a response to the external financial forces of the prospective payment system, contract bidding, and discounted rates from hospitals. For physicians, it is fee screens, utilization reviews, capitation payments, and discounted fees for services. In a fundamental way, the culture of medical care has changed in adapting to the new environment. Previously shared hospital and medical care values and beliefs are no longer realistic in today's environment of scarce resources.

New Ethical Concerns

Current ethical concerns differ from previous ethical issues in medical care. From the time of the Hippocratic Oath to the institution of a patient's bill of rights, ethical codes have defined the responsibilities and obligations of medicine and health care organizations toward patients. When physicians make an investment, whether in the stock market or a joint venture, they expect to earn a profit from their investment. If the investment is in a publicly traded stock, personal decisions of the physician-stockholder have no effect on dividends. But in local joint ventures, physician-investors can substantially affect a return on investment by ordering unnecessary tests and procedures and referring patients to a medical service in which they are shareholders.

In the recent past, physicians worked together to eliminate the unethical practices of ghost surgery and fee splitting. The Medicare program further protected patient interests by prohibiting various forms of kickbacks through defining fraud and abuse practices. In addition, many hospitals have adopted conflict of interests policies to prevent director and employee abuse of authority. Yet, some unethical corporate practices have escaped accountability.

Now emerging is a view that hospitals and physicians are placing financial motives and providers' economic concerns ahead of patient concerns. The public views medical care as a service to society, which only secondarily provides an economic benefit to physicians and hospitals.

Patients are becoming concerned. Reports in newspaper articles and congressional testimony have provided examples of excessive testing, unnecessary medical procedures, higher prices, and excessive profits, all affecting the public's trust in medical care. However, the true extent to which new medical care joint ventures may have abused the public interest is unknown.

Rationalizing Ethical Issues

The reasons used to justify investment in joint ventures vary. The usual reasons hospitals cite are the development of new revenue sources to offset Medicare and Medicaid payment shortfalls, the protection of existing market share, or the expansion of local market share. Physicians explain their joint venture investments as providing a higher quality service than previously available, replacing a similar hospital service with which they were dissatisfied, adding a new medical service to the community, or developing new income sources because the economic future of medical practice is increasingly uncertain.

Both hospitals and physicians explain their investments as good business sense, legal, and comparable to commercial firms investing in new business ventures. Overlooked, and unmentioned, is the traditional medical ethic that the patient's interests are primary and ahead of any personal interests of a physician or hospital.

The current wave of enthusiasm for joint ventures ignores society's long held viewpoint that medical care is more than a business. Society expects a higher standard of responsibility and accountability in medical care than from a business. The opportunity for a business to take advantage of a customer is typically limited by competition, honesty in advertising requirements, and a buyer's knowledge of the product or service. In contrast, a physician exercises discretionary medical judgment for treatments, procedures, and charges for these services without patients being able to judge either necessity or price.

Both physicians and hospitals have a higher calling than a business firm. Ethical physicians have a concern for the health and well-being of their patients, one that is responsive to a patient's individual needs and of more importance than the physician's personal needs. Ethical hospitals have a primary concern for the health status and well-being of their communities and patients, as well as a desire to be responsive to physician clinical directives.

The rush into joint ventures for additional revenue or as a competitive market strategy has modified the ethical standards of health care. This is not a new issue for the health care field. The American College of Surgeons created the Hospital Standardization Program because surgeons were concerned about medical ethics. They defined a physician's relationship to a hospital as separate and distinct from hospital employees by creating an organized, separate medical staff. They thought this arrangement was necessary to prevent patient care being compromised by hospitals.

There are differences in ethical standards for hospitals and physicians. Ethical conduct for a physician is defined as protecting and promoting the well-being of patients. It does not include a responsibility for the financial success of the hospitals, insurance carrier, or government medical program.

Hospitals have equally tough ethical standards to meet; they are expected to foster the well-being of both patients and the community and to ensure their own survival. Physicians are responsible for the diagnosis and treatment of patients, but the hospital cannot allow physicians to bankrupt the hospital in providing these services. Conflicts arise when financial survival is at stake as resources become more and more restricted.

Whether something is ethical or unethical depends on the ethical values of the individuals making these judgments. Some hospital executives or physicians justify their investment in joint ventures as necessary because of fee limitations for physicians and price caps for hospitals or because of utilization controls on both. Their concerns are over reduced incomes or revenues. Other hospital executives express opinions that freestanding imaging centers are unethical because they are sponsored by physicians who are also members of the hospital's medical staff. Physicians see it differently, expressing opinions that a hospital's efforts to stop the development of physician-sponsored centers of one kind or another are unethical. Both views are smokescreens for justifying personal opinions. Public displeasure has been expressed over managed care programs sponsored by hospitals and physicians. They are criticized as unethical because of the suspicion that hospitalized patients are discharged early or that needed diagnostic tests or treatment procedures are not ordered to reduce expenses and thereby increase profits.

Allegations of unethical practices by joint ventures have been made to justify opposition to them, whether or not there is in fact any abuse of ethical standards. Many joint ventures may be completely ethical in the conduct of their affairs but are viewed as unethical because of economic consequences for either hospitals or physicians. Most hospital CEOs and physicians are aware that ethical behavior is the bedrock of patient trust and essential to the public's belief in the health care system. Joint ventures, even those that are ethically operated, must avoid the appearance of unethical conduct.

An Ethical Dilemma

During the 1970s, only a few hospitals and physicians entered into economic relationships. Today, there is widespread concern that financial limitations will continue to be tightened, stimulating additional joint ventures. Heretofore, hospitals and physicians grudgingly accepted restrictive changes in payment systems and responded in a variety of interesting ways to maintain existing income levels. With the continuation of additional revenue restrictions, pressure to deviate from ethical standards will increase unless offset by the enforcement of Safe Harbor regulations.

The continued upward spiral of health care costs sets the stage for drastic revenue limitations. To remain completely ethical, hospitals and physicians will need deep pockets. As politicians, bureaucrats, industry and business leaders, and insurance executives adopt additional restrictions on their payments, the assumption seems to be that hospitals and physicians will continue to place their economic and practice freedoms secondary to their patient care responsibilities without questioning the price for being medically ethical. In the current environment, hospitals and physicians are in a quandary over this issue. As revenues are restricted, it is reasonable to expect hospitals and physicians to modify professional ethics. Ethical behavior is a two-way street and does not occur in a vacuum. Should Medicare combine hospital and physician payments as a way to improve the control of their payments to these providers, rage may be the response.

The actions of the federal government, insurance carriers, and business to restrict payments has created an ethical dilemma. Each payer has defined and limited its own responsibilities to the operational imperatives of their environment—Medicare to the direct costs of caring for the elderly and its affect on the federal deficit, insurance carriers to remaining competitive with other carriers, and business to remaining competitive in world markets. None of these viewpoints seriously considers the ultimate impact of their collective decisions on the financial stability of hospitals and physicians' willingness to provide the same standard of care.

In a larger sense, the gradual erosion of funding for indigents and the lack of broadly available health insurance coverage is an ethical matter and should be of concern to government, insurance carriers, and business. Instead, substantial portions of these responsibilities are being transferred by default to hospitals and physicians. Yet society continues to expect to receive needed medical care on demand even when payments are inadequate, denied, or not available to providers.

This lack of fairness by those responsible for paying health care bills, coupled with the public's expectations for quality medical care, creates the environment for joint ventures. There has been no demonstrable concern for the financial well-being of medical care providers. In a nutshell, utilitarianism has been the guiding principle, and payers have ignored equity for hospitals and physicians.

The Future

Unresponsive or irresponsible practices by government and business payers do not justify either the appearance of unethical practice or its actual occurrence in medical care. Medical relationships must provide for an ethical economic climate that protects patient interests. At the very least, joint ventures create a public suspicion and raise questions about the extent to which patients can trust that medical services are appropriate, necessary, and competitively priced.

Whenever unethical or questionable joint venture practices become public, all joint ventures become suspect, and public officials react by proposing legislation to eliminate questionable practices. Such proposals are often poorly defined and create unnecessary difficulties for ventures that are ethical. Safe harbors are a move in the desired direction but are unclear in definition.

As hospital bottom lines shrink and physician fees are restricted, joint ventures may continue to increase even though recent experience has shown that many such ventures have not been financially successful. As operating experience grows, it is likely that more of these ventures may become profitable. If partnerships between hospitals and physicians increase, then a way must be found to assure the public that these operations are ethical and are concerned with patient care and only less so with the pocketbooks of the providers of the service. In this case, safe harbors are a definite step in the right direction.

In 1985, Congress enacted Medicare fraud and abuse legislation to ensure a higher standard of ethical practice in medical care. In 1989, Congress amended this law. Medicare requirements sponsored by Representative Stark were enacted effective in 1992. The legislation prohibits referrals to medical services in which a physician has an ownership interest. This legislation does not protect non-Medicare patients, who constitute the bulk of referrals.

Not acknowledged by the current critics of medical practice ethics is that most hospitals and physicians have been sensitive to even the appearance of unethical behavior and have avoided involvement in joint business relationships. Physicians, as a group, have valued their medical integrity more than their financial well-being. Those physicians that continue to place medical integrity first will likely incur the largest losses in revenues by their refusal to compromise ethical values.

The existing regulatory environment allows business corporations and practitioners to take advantage of the unregulated medical marketplace for their own benefit. Ethically concerned hospitals and physicians who chose not to participate will be the financial losers. The Medicare Fraud and Abuse Act and the Stark bill do not prohibit the full range of potential ways to exploit patients. Creative medical entrepreneurs are alive and well, though in a minority. Most hospitals and physicians are ethical and will continue to maintain their standards.

Adhering to ethical medical standards is not the totality of ethical concerns for physicians and hospitals. Medical care is only one dimension of an individual's ethical conduct; physicians are parents, citizens, and community participants. Hospitals, as corporations, have a multiplicity of obligations to all levels of government and the judicial system, commercial obligations, and an obligation to be a model of the corporate community in a city.

It is the multiple ethical expectations that lead to conflicting ethical behavior. Ethical standards are manifestations of moral principles that serve as day-to-day guides for determining personal and corporate behavior in the daily environment. As payments decrease for medical care services, modifications of traditional medical ethics can be expected to occur. Existing ethics will be sidestepped or gradually modified to accommodate the new realities.

The issue is not one of change but rather whether change will occur from external forces or be internally driven by medical practitioners. Fundamental to any change is the protection needed to ensure that discretionary medical care judgments remain physician decisions. Protecting a physician's discretionary medical care decisions also provides the opportunity to exploit this freedom. Joint ventures provide a financial vehicle for profit at the expense of medical ethics. If traditional ethical standards of medical care are important to society, then they must be protected from all forms of abuse.

To continue to maintain traditional medical ethics requires the establishment of severe restraints, including a total ban on interlocking hospital and physician relationships and physician group to physician group investment arrangements. Safe harbors may ultimately reach this point.

An Alternative Approach

An accreditation program might be an acceptable way of maintaining public confidence. To be meaningful, an accreditation organization would need to demonstrate to the public that its program is objective and meaningful and that certification ensures ethical standards of operation. Even though standards for making such certifications are ethical, the appropriateness of the preliminary diagnosis, the medical history, and the referring physicians' comments might be used.

Excessive profits would be elusive to define and affected by fluctuating volumes, markups by test and procedure, and other variables. At best, expert judgment could only identify gross abuses. If arbitrary guides were developed for use, they would most likely be either too strict or too loose in any individual application. Certification would need both a medical and a financial audit by a respected independent organization; however, none exist.

Rapidly increasing medical care costs will sooner or later force the adoption of a new approach to providing medical care and paying for it. Most often proposed is a fixed fee system of paying physicians and the elimination of fee-for-service practice. Hospitals are likely to receive reduced DRG payments in inclusive per diem payments for all services.

Medical ethics are often the basis of laws, regulations, and common-law judgments that reinforce values or modify current practice. In Massachusetts, physicians are mandated to accept Medicare patients or risk the loss of their medical licenses. In Oregon, a formal medical care rationing system is being developed to identify reimbursable and nonreimbursable diagnoses and treatments based on anticipated outcomes. This step was backward since it does not guarantee access to medical care. In Massachusetts, a step forward was taken to ensure access for all. Both actions are responses to the financial realities of medical care; Oregon compromises access to medical care and Massachusetts compromises equity to the providers.

In the past, the providers' ability to shift costs made it possible for physicians and hospitals to absorb fee and income discounting by government and insurance carriers. As managed care programs expand, cost shifting decreases and physicians and hospitals lose revenue. As cost shifting is phased out, providers will be less concerned with medical ethics and more concerned with financial results.

It would be desirable to define future ways of avoiding the ethical pitfalls between patients and providers. Since there is no reasonable possibility that funding levels will improve rather than deteriorate further, the question of ethical values will grow in importance on the public's agenda. This increase in importance will lead to more legislative restrictions on economic relationships between hospitals and physicians with a growing concern over clinical and financial abuse of patients. Given sufficient time, society may gradually evolve a modified medical ethic that accommodates the financial reality. This decade will be a period of uncomfortable transition to a new medical ethic, as yet undefined. Medical ethics is an important societal issue and warrants serious attention by those who are concerned about the future of health care.

Notes

1. "$70 Consulting Fee Paid by a Texas Hospital to Physician for Each Patient Admitted," *Wall Street Journal*, 28 February 1989.
2. "Average Number of Tests Ordered by Physician Investor Was 6.23 Tests Per Patient and 3.76 for Non-Physician Investors," *Wall Street Journal*, 1 March 1989.
3. Ibid.

Part **III**

Meeting the Challenge
and Implementing Change

Chapter 7

Developing a Successful
Governing Board: The Basics

Since the turn of this century, U.S. hospitals have continued to evolve in a way that is unique among health care systems throughout the world. Unlike other health care systems that are federally owned or operated, the United States has three distinct types of hospitals: facilities owned by a unit of government, hospitals owned by for-profit investors, and not-for-profit hospitals owned and operated as philanthropic or religious institutions on behalf of a community. In the eyes of the public, not-for-profit hospitals have traditionally provided leadership for the industry. Academic centers have been noted for medical research, education, and cutting-edge technologies. Community hospitals have been noted for providing an excellent quality of care and being responsive to the health care needs of their communities.

To ensure responsiveness, hospital governing boards have been composed of outstanding local persons who voluntarily serve as trustees, giving freely of their time and energies on behalf of their communities. Representing the community has been the hallmark of trusteeship in hospitals and has been unchallenged for decades. Until economic competition entered the health care scene in 1983, there was little reason to believe that governing boards would ever need to change and adapt to new conditions.

Now external forces directly affect internal hospital operations and are forcing organizational reevaluations. Much of what has appeared in the literature on hospital governance has centered on the questions of size and composition but has not dealt with the relationship between hospitals and physicians—the one element that makes the hospital an organizational anomaly among all institutional forms of organization.

External forces, as demonstrated by the role of the federal government, have had severe effects on hospitals but have not led to modifications in hospital governance structures. Instead, hospitals have responded by developing multiple-type organizational structures—the local health care corporations with a mixture of not-for-profit and for-profit health-related companies. To date, many hospitals have not taken an analytical approach to the governance functions of a hospital but have assumed that existing board structure, in whatever form it is found, is the way it will probably be in the future.

Achieving a Superior Governing Board

Traditionally, governing boards of hospitals were modified by altering their structure and composition. The focus was more on form than on function. The degree to which governance functions were acceptably performed was a result of the form adopted. Board seats were either increased or decreased depending on the external demands, and board composition changed from time to time to more accurately reflect the representation the community desired. Changes in structure were considered sufficient to ensure improved board performance. Little, if any, attention was devoted to three other elements of successful board performance: the *competence* of individual board members, the *performance* of the governing board as an organizational unit of the hospital, and the *understanding* of health care sufficient to make sound decisions. These four elements,

Competence
Understanding
Performance
Structure

are all part and parcel of developing superior hospital governing boards.

Competence

Attention has recently been given to the question of competence in addition to the subject of structure. It is still regarded as a sensitive issue because of the long-established tradition of having community-minded citizens volunteering their services as board members. Improved competence begins with a selection process, with the first step a definition of the criteria required for board membership. Criteria are usually informal, subjectively determined in conversations that take place when a nominating committee gets together to discuss appointments and reappointments. Preferably, there should be an effective selection process that starts with having written criteria that are discussed, analyzed, and redrafted into a document that is regarded as realistic, substantial, and meaningful. It is the first step in an evaluation process.

Once criteria are defined, the selection process can begin in earnest. A list of potential candidates can be developed for both the immediate future and also for later consideration. Nominees need to know they are being considered and should be placed on a board membership mailing list if they show interest. Persons being considered need to understand their performance as a board member will be evaluated annually. The format of the annual evaluation should be given to them if it is available. The message communicated is that the business of hospital governance is all business and that individual performance will be evaluated annually.

In publicly owned hospitals, with board members appointed by local governmental bodies, this same process can be followed. City leaders and county commissioners should be given the criteria for guidance in selecting board members. When board members are appointed, the same process of indoctrination that nonpublic hospitals use should be followed.

Understanding

For some unknown reason, hospital chief executives have typically assumed that newly elected board members do not need much time to learn about the health care field and that a general orientation to the community's problems will suffice as a backdrop for making hospital decisions. Reading material sent out prior to board meetings, along with a subscription to an appropriate journal, largely make up the material devoted to developing a trustee's understanding of the health field. One often hears a long-time governing board member remark that it takes two to three years before any real understanding of health care develops.

An important question in the fast-changing health care environment is, How much specific knowledge about the health care field is needed before a board member can effectively function as part of the governance structure? Another question is, How should this information be acquired? Given the peculiarities of an industry where the medical staff is an organizational entity, where the definition of fraud and abuse are very different from commercial definitions, where DRGs pay for 44 percent nationally of all inpatient days of care, and where malpractice liability and antitrust are serious threats, the potential damage that uninformed board members can cause gives added weight to the necessity of having informed board members. Even when a selection process is well developed for screening, evaluating, and selecting potential board members, an organized plan to develop understanding about health care is needed.

When a person has been identified as suitable for board membership, developing a minimum acceptable level of understanding of health care is the second step. A combination of methods may be employed to achieve these results. After nomination for a board seat and being placed on a mailing list for materials sent to the governing board, there is an additional requirement. Before attending their first board meeting, a new board member should be required to attend an orientation program of several hours. Once on the governing board, an annual board retreat is helpful, as well as attendance at trustee seminars conducted by hospital associations.

One of the major reasons governing boards have paid little attention to the need for continuing knowledge about trends in the health care field is that this responsibility has been left up to the chief executive. Preferably, the chairperson of the governing board should be the individual responsible for these activities. The chairperson sets the tone for the board and should take the initiative for ensuring that board members have appropriate and up-to-date knowledge of the health field trends.

Performance

The third ingredient of a successful governing board is an ability to arrive at timely and appropriate decisions. It is the mix of talents on a board that enables all relevant information, experience, and viewpoints to be brought to bear on subjects under discussion.

Performance is the sum total of the individual board members' collective wisdom around the board table. It is arriving at balanced judgments, often from among differing viewpoints. The chairperson of the board faces the same kind of problem as does the conductor of a symphony orchestra. All parts must be kept in balance and one section cannot be permitted to dominate the entire orchestra, or the result is less than acceptable. The chief executive functions like the concert master of the orchestra, providing leadership in support of the conductor.

Like an orchestra member, the contribution of each board member is important, but it is the sum total of all of their efforts that determines the degree of success the governing board attains.

Structure

The fourth ingredient of an effective board is its organizational structure. While functions to be performed should dictate the form of structure needed, it is more likely to be the other way around, that functions have to be adapted to fit the existing form of organization. This is understandable but detrimental since the structure of a typical hospital governing body was developed when the hospital corporation was originally incorporated. The number of board members and the type of representation incorporated on the board were determined at its inception and often remain locked in place with only minor modifications. Over time, a governance structure becomes less and less relevant to its functions because of the accumulated changes that take place in the external environment.

Eventually, the organizational form continues to dictate the rate at which decisions are reached and who can make them while the quality of decisions and effective governance become secondary to maintaining an existing structure. In past years, with the health care field stable and revenues ample, the proper functioning of the board was not a matter of great concern. As revenues have decreased and economic competition has grown, it has become important to rebalance the relationship between the form and the function of governance. Like in all successful organizations, the functions to be performed must dictate the size and composition of the structure of governance.

Conclusions

In times of economic stress, with the future highly unpredictable, the role of governance is crucial to success. While it may not ultimately determine the survivability of a hospital, it may ultimately determine its failure. The four requirements of a successful board—competence, understanding, performance, and structure—are crucial in times of severe stress.

All too often, when the role of governance is reviewed, the focus is almost always on structure. An assumption is made that if a properly developed structure is put in place, that is all that is needed to ensure that the governing board will be effective and competent. That some board members do not do their homework, that others lack relevant knowledge and experience, and that still other board members see their role as being of more importance than that of anyone else associated with the health care organization reflect a total lack of understanding what is required in organizationally traumatic times. Yet when one looks beyond structure at the three other aspects of successful governance—competence, understanding, and performance—it is evident that substantive decisions can only be reached when all four ingredients are given equal weight.

To look at all four elements seriously and analytically requires objectivity and courage from members of governance. It also requires that board members believe that the overall performance of governance is more important than the interests of individual directors. Successful hospital boards must be willing to experience some discomfort to attain the levels of performance that are necessary to meet the future demands of the health care system.

To restructure governance for better performance requires an understanding of the changes occurring in health
care and how to refit the organization to accommodate
these new realities. The remaining chapters in this book address some of the difficult issues related to the four elements of successful governance. The two questionnaires in
the appendix may be used both to educate governing members about their leadership role and to gather their input
and ideas regarding ways to improve leadership.

Chapter 8

The Competent Board: Voluntary or Enterprise?

One perplexing problem in the health care field today is what to do about governing boards in voluntary not-for-profit hospitals and in local not-for-profit health care corporations. In private, many chief executives of these organizations single out governance as their most intractable problem, pointing out it is more often a hindrance and not of much assistance in developing policy. On the other hand, members of governing boards report that chief executives can be too quick to forget community interests vis à vis a hospital's interests and the board's essential role to be mindful of that community interest. Given these differences in perspective, the question is not which is right and which is wrong but rather what should governance be like in the future. Should it change? If so, how? Do board members need to reexamine the traditional philosophy of trusteeship in light of the changes taking place in the health care field?

Professional health care consultants see a need to undertake such a reexamination but are of the opinion that most members of governing boards are unwilling to seriously review, evaluate, or significantly alter their philosophy on the role of governing boards. The basic reason for serving on a not-for-profit health care governing authority seems to be so deeply rooted in individuals serving in this capacity that they do not even want to consider any other approach or concept. In essence, the rationale appears to be, As a good citizen, I am fulfilling my civic responsibility by serving on this board. I do this on behalf of my friends and neighbors, representing the community interests in this important social activity as their agent. In doing so, I expect no pay and give of my time to serve the public good.

Under such philosophical constraints, examining the role of governance in not-for-profit health care organizations becomes a highly charged, sensitive issue. A critical look at the beliefs and principles that have been the bedrock of trusteeship for decades is fraught with emotional overtones and becomes difficult to examine in a thoughtful, objective manner. Nevertheless, it is a subject whose time has come, and a public dialogue is needed.

The Traditional Voluntary Board: Representing Community Interests

Hospitals began as endeavors of religious groups who saw the need to minister to the physical well-being of people as well as to their spiritual needs. This tradition of voluntary service to the needy was expanded as the medical armamentarium grew and was able to cope with a wider and wider range of illness. By the 1920s, hospitals were acknowledged as institutions where the public should go to get well. This development was important because society had moved from an agrarian economy to one where the majority of the population lived in urban areas and were wage earners. Being able to get well was crucial to earning a living, and hospitals were pivotal in healing people. Hospital governing boards recognized this relationship and saw their role as an important civic responsibility in keeping with traditions that extended back to the Middle Ages. Serving one's fellow citizens by serving on a hospital board was something to be proud of; representing the community in this activity grew into one of the most important roles one could undertake as a demonstration of civic involvement.

When Blue Cross was born in the late 1920s and rapidly developed into the dominant prepayment mechanism to finance hospital care, it buttressed the concept of representative governance in hospitals. Blue Cross, in its early stage, based premiums on community rating (versus experience rating) and paying all hospitals full operating costs, whether they were high-cost or low-cost hospitals. Since Blue Cross was the main source of revenue and typically paid on a cost reimbursement basis, governing boards were unrestrained in their desire to respond totally to the community interest, reinforcing the concept of representative governance. When Medicare and Medicaid were enacted in 1965, they also adopted the cost reimbursement method of paying hospitals, which also reinforced this concept.

Until the early 1980s, when economic competition appeared on the hospital scene, representative governance was never questioned; it was simply the way all not-for-profit health care corporations were organized. It was understood that governing board members were trustees and that their responsibility was to hold the community and public interest in trust. They acted on behalf of the community. No serious thought was given to being an enterprise board that would put the interests of the hospital first and the interests of the community second.

Being a board member was a position of trust, and the personal integrity of each member had to be well above reproach. The level of integrity that was expected required board members to donate to their time and to receive no compensation for performing governance duties. As outsiders to health care, it would seem appropriate that they should lean more heavily on the chief executive for policy judgments. Typically, they did not, because they saw themselves as the interpreters of community interests and therefore as responsible for making the decisions involved in governing the hospital, even though they lacked industry knowledge and experience.

From this perspective, board members usually viewed their role as seeing to it that the health care corporation or hospital operated cost effectively. To bring this about, governing boards typically met monthly to review operating reports. As conservators, they are concerned that the assets of the corporation not be dissipated but used to the best advantage. To do this effectively, board members need an in-depth knowledge of the operations they are reviewing, which is usually lacking. Having in-depth knowledge is of particular importance in a hospital where the quality of patient care is a major component of how well the hospital is operating.

Because quality of care cannot be measured by numbers but largely depends on observation by competent professionals, it becomes an elusive criterion to most governing board members. Yet month after month, year after year, board members review financial and statistical data without having any solid basis for arriving at judgments about hospital operations. Little if any thought is given to whether or not this is an effective exercise for the board to undertake.

In the past, reviewing the operating statistics of a health care organization was appropriate when revenues were substantially generated from cost reimbursement sources. It has become less and less relevant as economic competition and negotiated prices have become accepted practices. To survive in an economically competitive environment, a different orientation is needed and the traditional guidelines of a not-for-profit community hospital governing board need to be reexamined. Until this decade, governing boards were philosophically wedded to the following ideals: the best possible care, the lowest possible cost, and responsiveness to community need. In an economically competitive environment in a mature industry with too much capacity, hospitals that cling to these traditional beliefs will inevitably encounter serious financial consequences.

Defining community interests

A not-for-profit hospital governing board that puts the community interests above all other considerations might assume that by doing so the hospital will continue to survive indefinitely in the future. The reasoning behind such a stance is a belief that, as a community agency in which no individual board member has a pecuniary interest, the worthwhileness of the activity will continue to be recognized and therefore the hospital's longevity assured. The difficulty in an economically competitive environment is that the traditional breadth of commitment of the not-for-profit hospital is so broad that it cannot be fulfilled without jeopardizing the financial stability of the organization. The more economically competitive a marketplace becomes, the greater the necessity for having a hospital-focused commitment.

Not-for-profit health care boards rarely directly define the elements of community interests. Board members view their responsibility as making the hospital responsive to the community, which is the purpose for which a not-for-profit corporate structure was adopted. Because the legal structure is a corporation, the board unthinkingly assumes all of its decisions are, per se, in the community's interest. In this form of organization, it is never necessary to define the community interests; anything decided by the governing board becomes the community's interest.

The belief seems to be that the spirit of volunteerism is embodied in its not-for-profit status and that as long as it remains alive, that will ultimately ensure the survival of the hospital or health care corporation. Representative governance is viewed as fundamental to the institution's role in society. Emotional blinders prevent asking, Can voluntary, not-for-profit hospitals survive if they continue to rely on representative governance in an increasingly economically competitive climate? Avoiding this question will not make it go away, but it may lead to unanticipated consequences.

Under representative governance the primary interest is in answering the health care needs of the community; all other concerns are of lesser importance. Yet in a competitive environment, the primary interest has to be organizational effectiveness if a health care corporation is going to survive in a mature industry with excess capacity. Under existing conditions, financial matters become primary. Those with strong allegiances to the concept of voluntary, not-for-profit health care organizations may disagree as they see this shift as placing too much emphasis on dollars and not enough on cooperation and coordination with other not-for-profit organizations all striving to serve community need. Yet to give financial matters only a secondary position is an invitation to financial disaster, which would render the hospital unable to serve anybody.

Voluntary, community-minded hospital trustees might not recognize the financial dangers that now exist because of their lack of in-depth knowledge and experience in the industry, which can lead them to make decisions based on the conditions of today rather than on what is likely to occur in the health field in three to five years. Trustees are aware that other nearby hospitals now have to be regarded as competitors and as predators on their share of the market, but their community orientation leads them still to prefer cooperation and coordination with other hospitals.

In a climate dominated by economic competition, the hospital that puts community interests first will eventually be providing patient services that no other hospital will offer because of the financial disincentives. In the future, the "community first" hospital may be faced with bankruptcy or becoming a charity hospital, receiving most of its funds from a tax-supported body for providing care to patients that other hospitals are unwilling to provide for financial reasons. Stated in another way, those hospitals with an eye on the economics of health care will skim off the paying patients leaving the partial and no-pay patients to the hospital that decides to focus on service to the community.

As Medicare payments become more restrictive and HMOs grow, the importance of economic considerations will become greater. With an increasingly loud voice, representative-type boards of not-for-profit health care organizations will likely argue that their hospitals are being treated unfairly since they seek only to serve community interests. They may attempt to level the playing field for health care through legislative redress. Such an approach is a time-consuming, lengthy process with questionable outcomes.

Not-for-profit governing boards organized on some basis other than representation will respond to these circumstances differently. Top priority will be given to looking for avenues that enhance market share in those patient categories where revenues exceed the costs of providing the services.

Enterprise Boards: Responding to Economic Constraints

As a result of the tightening of the economic screws on hospital revenues, many voluntary not-for-profit hospitals will be converted into parent-subsidiary organizational structures in a search for alternative revenue sources. The hospital will remain a 501(c)(3) corporation, the parent will likewise be not-for-profit, but additional for-profit subsidiaries will be created for generating revenues from other inpatient sources.

Where parent-subsidiary models have been put in place, for-profit subsidiaries are still of minor importance in most cases. As they grow, they may come to equal the hospital as an economic entity and thereby diminish the importance of the not-for-profit activities. The status accorded the outside directors of the for-profit subsidiaries will correspondingly increase. As substantial profits increase, the payment of annual honorariums and payments for attending committee meetings is likely to be initiated in keeping with the practices in other for-profit corporations. This will set up a catch-22 situation where those outside directors serving on the not-for-profit boards of the hospital and the parent organization will view themselves as being treated unfairly. It is unlikely that the answer will be to cease paying the outside directors of the for-profit subsidiaries but rather to commence paying the trustees like amounts.

The argument most frequently put forth against paying trustees for their services is that the amount paid would not come close to matching what they can earn in their career positions. While this is true, this line of reasoning overlooks fundamental characteristics of hospital trustees. They are responsible persons, and the payment for their services, no matter how little it may be, symbolizes their responsibility to the hospital. The payment of a fee can change the seriousness with which they approach the obligations of directorship and trusteeship.

Defining volunteerism

When the not-for-profit community hospital converts to a health care corporation that is a combination of for-profit and not-for-profit activities with all board members paid annual honorariums, the question arises, What is volunteerism in the health field? The answer lies in defining volunteerism as something other than being an unpaid trustee.

To examine volunteerism it is useful to compare the operation of a for-profit hospital and a not-for-profit one. The difference between the two is not to be found in differing management techniques; they are the same in both. The for-profit hospital may initially stress the financial indicators to a greater extent, but as the revenue sources for all hospitals become more restrictive, both will emphasize finances to the same degree. The distinguishing characteristics lie elsewhere.

A comparison of the medical staffs of the two types reveals no differences. They are both organized in the same manner and are responsible in like manner for patient care. But many for-profit hospitals have both physicians and senior executives as governing board members. Boards composed of both insiders and outsiders are better able to assess quality of care issues than not-for-profit boards that exclude insiders.

By and large, outside members of hospital governing boards are not aware that the one and only purpose of an organized medical staff is to ensure patient safety. Many trustees do not view the medical staff as an integral part of the hospital organization. They tend to view the medical staff as separate and apart from the hospital because the majority of physicians are independent contractors and not employees of the hospital. Physicians are viewed as customers or clients because they decide when and where to hospitalize patients. Governing boards take pains not to upset them.

The result of this thinking is that the governing board treats the medical staff as an economic entity rather than as a mechanism for ensuring quality of care. This buttresses the physicians' notion that the role of a hospital is to support their economic interests or, at a minimum, to be neutral with respect to them. All too often, board members buy into this line of reasoning. Both board members and physicians tend to believe that the medical staff bylaws document is a contract between two equal parties rather than an agreement defining how the overall organization and a component part of the organization will relate to each other. (The medical staff organization and bylaws are discussed in Chapter 9.)

Outside board members often are of the opinion that a medical staff actually functions in the way it is defined in the medical staff bylaws. Experienced hospital executives appreciate that that is rarely the case. Because they are independent as private practitioners, many physicians believe that the less structure there is to the organization, the better the place is for them to center their hospital activities.

In spite of these long-standing difficulties, a serious effort has never developed among not-for-profit governing boards to rethink the board–medical staff relationship and to propose creative ways for achieving a more productive organizational structure.

In the typical hospital, 20 percent of the medical staff members admit 80 percent of the patients, yet all physicians expect to be treated as equals by the hospital even though their relationships to it are unequal. As economic competition between hospitals grows and financial concerns about survivability increase, the bond between the 20 percent who are substantial admitters and the hospital needs to be strengthened. Quid pro quos that are specifically tailored to each individual relationship should be developed. Two factors are important. A hospital needs to determine and enforce its own standards of patient care and should expect all patients requiring hospitalization to be admitted to its facility. In return, the hospital should be receptive to the needs of the client physicians and assist in enhancing their practices. This may include spending advertising dollars, allocating space, and providing unique equipment. The two parties should be bound together by contract in a meaningful economic relationship that benefits both of them. All hospitals need this relationship, but it may be difficult to achieve because of the complexity of physician-to-physician relationships as well as the hospital-physician relationship. Those institutions that are successful in developing and maintaining such contractual relationships will be the leaders in the field by the turn of the next century.

Volunteerism cannot be defined in terms of the internal operations of the hospital or the organization of the medical staff. When the governing boards of not-for-profit hospitals and for-profit hospitals are compared, there are decided differences in terms of philosophy, composition, role, and operation.

In a study conducted by the Wyatt Company, 337 health care organizations were queried.[1] The average not-for-profit governing board size was reported to be 13.9 members with a tendency for the size of the board to increase with the number of hospital beds in the system. Terms of membership on the typical board were three years with those selected representing a cross section of community, business, and professional elites. Physicians were represented on 86 percent of the boards included in the study, while chief executives were represented on 58 percent. The number of other insiders was not reported. Seventy-one percent indicated they had separate foundation boards engaged in fund-raising.

Our personal experience in working with a large number of community, not-for-profit, voluntary hospitals is that governing boards usually believe it is necessary to control the production-type operations of the institution to carry out their mandate. To avoid using excessive amounts of any individual board member's time, a large number of board committees are created to oversee various aspects of the hospital operation and to recommend actions to the full board.

To ensure that committee activities are coordinated with the work of the full board, considerable chunks of senior management time are required. Time devoted to governance activities means less time for directing operational activities. In many instances, the chief executive of a not-for-profit hospital devotes between 25 and 50 percent of work time to governance activities. The question whether this investment of time and effort by all those involved is worth the results obtained is seldom if ever raised or evaluated. Board members consider these meetings as part of their responsibilities. It is assumed that because the executives' time is spent on governance, it supersedes any other activity. No one considers whether this is a desirable way of conducting the affairs of a hospital in today's economy.

The amount of time that a chief executive spends on governance with a representative-type board is often a function of its size. The larger the board, the more committees it is likely to create. Chairpersons of voluntary boards often take the position that it is unfair to ask only a portion of the board membership to serve on board committees, so they create enough committees so that all members are included. Little thought is given to the additional amount of executive time required to staff these activities or of the lengthening of the decision-making chain that takes place. Looked at objectively, the primary role of senior management appears to be to serve the governance function, rather than for governance to serve the purposes of the hospital. Boards rarely ask themselves if they are requiring too much of a chief executive's time.

As a rule, voluntary boards believe that community interests are primary and that hospital interests are secondary. In contrast, board members view the chief executive as having the hospital as his primary concern but giving community interests second place. The voluntary board sees recommendations from the chief executive in the light of its primary responsibility of protecting the community interests rather than from the perspective of the impact on the hospital operation. This approach to evaluating recommendations places the chief executive in a master-servant relationship to the voluntary governing board. Even in hospitals where the chief executive has demonstrated outstanding competence over two or three decades, the relationship remains.

Voluntary board members are often of the opinion that it is more important to appreciate the community's interests than it is to be knowledgeable about hospital matters. Yet in a mature industry with excess capacity and increasing constraints on inpatient revenues, the overriding concerns of these board members are finance, internal operations, and adherences to policy, all of which require in-depth knowledge of hospital operations. In for-profit health care corporations, local and corporate managements make these types of decisions. Corporate boards concentrate on other matters.

The distinguishing characteristic of a voluntary, not-for-profit hospital is in its basic philosophy. Profits from hospital operations, philanthropic gifts, and profits from related activities are either plowed back into capital expenditures or used to underwrite patient care. As third party payers increasingly restrict hospital revenues, forcing a reduction in cost-shifting activities, the importance of the not-for-profit corporate structure for hospitals will gain in public acceptability. They will continue to adhere to their basic philosophy of providing care to the financially disadvantaged as well as vigorously competing for other categories of patients. Even though its reason for being continues, the not-for-profit, voluntary hospital needs to rethink the governance function.

Lessons from corporate governing boards

Other industries provide a model that needs to be examined and evaluated.[2] Enterprise boards tend to be small in number, have few committees, and meet infrequently. Their primary responsibilities are to be the corporate conscience, to discourage thinking in stereotypes, to stimulate, to counsel, and to support the chief executive. Enterprise boards periodically evaluate the chief executive's performance, but they are more concerned about issues of strategy, new opportunities, marketing conditions, trends, and the regulatory climate. As a result, time devoted to a review of operations is minimal, the main interest being positioning within the industry.

Meetings of enterprise boards are most often held quarterly, each meeting lasting six to seven hours, with the bulk of the time focused on strategy. The outcomes of these meetings do not require consensus. New programs are discussed, diverse opinions expressed, tough questions asked, but the chief executive is expected to move ahead on his or her plans. Consensus is not important. Board members are paid an annual honorarium and per diem amounts for participation in committee meetings. The chief executive is a key member of the board of directors and has a collegial relationship with its members and the chairperson, since they are on a relatively equal plane. More often than not, the chairperson and the chief executive are of one mind about most problems since they have in-depth industry experience and knowledge. Together they plan the board agenda and determine the outcome they desire—decision, advice, briefing, problem identification, or problem solving. An enterprise board's main function is to be a think tank that acts as a sounding board for the chief executive.

Since the conditions of the marketplace are in constant flux, the membership of the board rapidly changes. Knowledgeable outsiders who have insights that can contribute to the welfare of the corporation are brought onto the board. Some inside board members may be rotated on and off of the board as the expertise requirements change. These changes enable the corporation to survive and prosper in its marketplace.

Of course, the objective is the same for a not-for-profit community hospital. The only significant difference is that any profits that are realized are plowed back into providing services the community needs. In return for not taking out profits, the states and federal government permit these corporations to be tax exempt. The only characteristic that differentiates a not-for-profit corporation from a for-profit one is how profits are used. Because of this similarity, it is possible to reorganize a representative-type governing board into an enterprise board.

Would an enterprise board express the community will and serve its interests as well as a representative board? How this question is answered depends on what is likely to occur in the health care field over the remaining years of this century. If cost reimbursement was restored as the dominant source of hospital revenue, community interests would again become primary and a resurgence of representative-type governing boards could take place. All decisions could again be based on doing good for the community, knowing that the revenues to cover all the activities would be forthcoming. Concern about the financial viability of the hospital would not be a factor; it would be assured because of the financing mechanism used to pay hospitals.

On the other hand, if the trend continues toward pricing mechanisms and negotiated contracts for hospital services, then all hospitals will be forced to give community interests a secondary position and to pay primary attention to their financial viability. A hospital that is not financially viable will find itself unable to provide any services to the community. The choice is not between for-profit and not-for-profit; either form of corporate organization can be effective. Rather, the choice lies in adopting a governance structure that best meets the demands of the times in which hospitals find themselves.

Representative-type boards and the enterprise board are contrasted in Table 8.1. Given these differences, a choice needs to be made. It seems appropriate to ask oneself, Which organizational model should be used given the existing climate? If you had to bet on one or the other, which one would you prefer?

If the choice is in favor of moving to the enterprise board model, the ability of the chief executive to adapt to a significant role change comes into question. In all probability the mortality rate among chief executives of representative-type governing boards will rise. Those who have spent two or more decades living under the master-servant relationship that dominates the not-for-profit scene are apt to be unable to make the transition. They have spent too many years learning and honing the political skills required to

Table 8.1   Comparison of Representative Boards and Enterprise Boards

Representative Board	Enterprise Board
Board Characteristics	
Community driven	Industry driven
Large boards	Small boards
Many committees	Few committees
Service ethic	Service and business ethic
Slow decision making	Rapid decision making
Slow board turnover	Rapid board turnover
Production oriented	Consumer oriented
10–12 board meetings annually	4–6 board meetings annually
2–3-hour board meetings	6–7-hour board meetings
Limited authority delegated	Wide authority delegated
Lacking in health industry experience	Health industry well represented
Overriding Concerns	
Finance	Strategy
Internal operations	New opportunities
Adherence to policy	Quality assurance
Board Member Characteristics	
Trustee	Director
Conservator	Risk taker
Unpaid	Paid
Attends more meetings	Attends fewer meetings
Concerned with fundraising generation	Concerned with revenue
Lacks full understanding of industry complexity	Appreciates industry complexity
Inability to evaluate quality of care	Ability to evaluate quality of care
Chief Executive Characteristics	
Nonvoting member of board	Voting member of board
Servant of the board	Colleague of board members
No employment contract	Employment contract
Agent of the board	Leader of the board

Continued

Table 8.1 Continued

Representative Board	Enterprise Board
Spends 25–50 percent of time on governance	Spends 10 percent of time on governance
Not involved in board selection	Key in board selection
Accountability lacks definition	Accountability is clear cut

survive in the representative-type organizational model and will be unable to shift to a new role. The techniques and skills needed to manage the internal operations and medical staff relationships remain the same in either model. The difference lies in the relationships to the governing board.

Those who are presently at the second level of health care organizations have an advantage. By and large, they are more recent MBA graduates (health care concentrations or the equivalent) and possess more up-to-date analytical skills. Secondly, their manipulative skills are not as finely honed as those of the chief executive so they do not have to retrain their thought patterns. Second-level executives carry less baggage in this regard and have less of an adjustment to make. The management skills remain unaltered, but major changes are required in leadership skills. An enterprise board favors a chief executive who exhibits an entrepreneurial spirit and a willingness to take risks. A chief executive who is averse to taking risks will not survive with an enterprise board.

Some believe that typical chief executives in voluntary hospitals will not be able to make the necessary adjustments because they have become too dependent for too long on their governing boards. What needs to be appreciated is that they have not yet had an opportunity in their careers to demonstrate any other type of behavior. The number that can rise to the occasion is simply unknown. Most chief executives have chafed at the behaviors they have had to adopt. Many may be too optimistic about what they can accomplish if they work with an enterprise board. The odds for survival seem to favor those who are not beyond midcareer. Their graduate education embodied management theory and organization, so they understand what is required in an enterprise model and lack only practice in putting it into use.

The future of not-for-profit health care organizations favors those that critically review and analyze their strengths and weaknesses. The most careful look of all needs to be directed at the governance structure. This is not an easy task because of its sensitivity, but it is a needed step if the not-for-profit health care organization is to be alive and well in the coming decade. Viability depends partly on how well individual board members carry out their responsibilities. Individual performance needs to be measured. Recognizing this need, national associations have developed self-evaluation forms. This "toe in the water" approach avoids facing up to what is needed. A serious method for measuring individual performance is required.

Notes

1. *Practices of Boards of Directors/Trustees in the Health Care Industry*, (Fort Lee, NJ. Executive Compensation Services, subsidiary of Wyatt Co., 1986).
2. "A Moment of Opportunity—Transitioning from Trusteeship to Strategic Direction" (unpublished presentation by André L. Delbecq, at an Estes Park Faculty Retreat, July 1986, Sun Valley, Idaho).

Chapter 9

Understanding the Clinical Component: Criteria for Medical Staff Organization

One of the most frequent comments members of hospital governing boards make is that it takes them three years to really begin to understand the complexities of the hospital organization. Three factors contribute to this difficulty. Third parties typically pay for hospital services on behalf of the patient; Blue Cross, HMOs, commercial insurance, Medicare, and Medicaid—all have different formulas, quite unlike anything encountered in the business world. Another complexity is the social nature of the community hospital, operated as a not-for-profit entity providing for many of the health care needs of the community. And the most confusing of all is the medical staff organization composed of practicing physicians who operate under a set of medical staff bylaws and rules and regulations that govern their actions in the hospital and are approved by the governing board.

The purpose of medical staff bylaws is to ensure patient safety and define the organizational structure for making this possible. To be effective, the roles of the governing board, the medical executive committee, the clinical departmental chiefs of service and their departments, and the vice-president of medical affairs need to be defined in terms of responsibility, authority, and accountability. In addition, it is necessary to make these same determinations for the officers of the medical staff—the president, the vice-president or president elect, and the secretary-treasurer. If the functions of those who medically manage the medical staff and those who administratively manage the medical staff are comingled, it becomes even more important to carefully define responsibility, authority, and accountability.

Since the medical staff is an organizational substructure that is part of the total hospital, the general principles of organization theory apply. For example, the chief of a clinical department is responsible for maintaining the quality of medical care provided by the members of the department and must have the necessary authority to require compliance with departmental standards. If the authority to do the job is inadequate, the clinical chief cannot be held accountable for the results. Authority and responsibility must be balanced if accountability to the next higher organizational level is to be effectively enforced. The following criteria for medical staff organization explain the typical responsibilities, authority, and accountability of members of the medical substructure and provide a context for understanding medical staff bylaws.

The Governing Board

The governing board is ultimately accountable for everything that happens in the hospital. It finally approves and adopts all policies, including those pertaining to medical care. It receives recommendations from the medical executive committee concerning medical staff bylaws, rules, regulations, and standards of care but cannot delegate its authority to alter or modify them. A summary report of professional care activities designed to permit comparisons with the standard of care established by the hospital should be submitted regularly to the governing board.

The governing board, on the recommendations of the medical executive committee, appoints all members of clinical departments, the chiefs of service who are the heads of clinical departments (see below), and the chairperson of the medical executive committee. The governing board should establish criteria for the eligibility of members of the medical staff for the position of chief of service to assist the clinical departments in making acceptable recommendations. The governing board appoints chiefs of each major clinical department to the medical executive committee. In addition, the committee recommends three members of the active staff for the board to appoint. These appointments may not be made from among those staff members who would be serving as staff officers (president, vice-president, or secretary-treasurer), since staff officers are elected by their peers to serve the best interests of the medical staff rather than the hospital as a whole.

The executive committee of the governing board should meet at least quarterly with the medical executive committee. The decisions reached at such meetings are subject to appropriate ratification before being effective.

The Medical Executive Committee

The medical executive committee is the authoritative body of the medical staff. It is accountable for the effectiveness of all medical care activities within the hospital. It formulates medical care policies for the medical staff and recommends timely action. The medical executive committee is the unit of the medical staff responsible for all matters of professional ethics and discipline. It may delegate this responsibility to the chiefs of service and hold them accountable. The medical executive committee recommends the organization, including departmentalization, of the medical staff and any changes that may be required from time to time. It regularly reviews the administrative and clinical performance of the chiefs of service. The chiefs should regularly submit summaries of the statistical data concerning the quality of care to the medical executive committee.

The size and composition of the medical executive committee should be determined by the governing board on the recommendation of the committee. Each major clinical department should be represented on the medical executive committee by the chief of service, whether or not any other member of the department is appointed to the committee. Members of the staff other than chiefs of service may be nominated to the governing board by the medical staff as a whole at an annual medical staff business meeting or by the medical executive committee at a meeting called for that purpose. The appointed clinical chiefs of service should comprise a majority of the Medical Executive Committee. The terms of appointment should be sequential so that a majority of committee members are retained at all times. The committee nominates a chairperson from among its own members. The president of the hospital or his or her designate (e.g., the medical director or the vice-president of medical affairs) should be an ex officio member of the committee.

The medical executive committee is responsible for the professional conduct of all members of the medical staff and for recommending medical staff bylaws, rules, and regulations to the governing board. It makes recommendations on all matters related to the care and treatment of patients and on medical education programs conducted in the hospital. It may advise the governing board through the board's chairperson on all activities pertaining to the welfare of the hospital. The medical executive committee reviews and recommends to the governing authority the credentials of those seeking appointment to the medical staff and evaluates medical care activities. It may delegate the review of credentials and medical care activities to the clinical departments. On the recommendation of the chiefs of services and on the basis of professional competence, the medical executive committee approves the extent of practice privileges for each member of the medical staff (see also below regarding the chiefs of services). It should be assured through appropriate reports, both formal and informal, that each clinical department regularly reviews the medical care its members give. It should also receive reports of all formal disciplinary activities within clinical departments.

The medical executive committee creates committees from time to time to carry out special functions. The function of these committees should be to investigate for, advise, and make recommendations to the medical executive committee.

Chiefs of Services

The chiefs of services are the heads of each clinical department. Each chief is responsible for implementing the actions of the medical executive committee within his or her department.

The chief holds all members of the staff practicing in the department accountable for meeting the professional standards of care established for the hospital. He or she may establish departmental standards that exceed the standards established for the hospital as a whole. The chief of service is also responsible for the professional conduct of all members of the medical staff in his or her department.

The chief of service enforces privilege limitations in the department. He or she regularly reviews the performance of all members of the medical staff in the department. The chief prepares a written review of the qualifications and privileges of each member of the department annually during the first five years of each appointment and triennially after that. He or she also reviews the performance of other members of the medical staff with practice privileges in the department on the same basis as members of the department. The chief recommends the departmental practice privileges for members of the medical staff and may reduce or suspend privileges whenever indicated, subject to prompt review by the medical executive committee.

The chief of service determines what matters department members should vote on. Statistical data concerning the professional activities in a department should be regularly reported to the chief of service.

The term of office of the chief of service should be three years, to permit the establishment of a stable and successful departmental program. The appointment should be contingent on membership on the medical staff of the hospital. Chiefs of services should be permitted to succeed themselves for one term if they are renominated at the completion of the appointment.

Clinical Departments

The work of the medical staff is conducted through organized clinical departments. Each member of the medical staff should be appointed to a specific department. Departmental meetings should be held at least monthly. At some hospitals, the members of a department nominate a chief of service to the governing authority.

All appointments should provide for reasonable tenure. Appointments other than to the courtesy staff should be for one year for the first five years and biannually after that. Courtesy staff appointments, for practitioners who occasionally admit patients, should be for one year, renewable annually. Emeritus staff appointments, which may be given for long and outstanding service, should be of indefinite tenure, the performance of such emeritus staff members being subject to annual review. If the medical executive committee requests, staff members must submit to a physical evaluation by a member of the medical staff the staff member selects from a list of medical members chosen by the medical executive committee.

The appointment of each staff member should provide for clearly delineated privileges, not only in the department to which the member is appointed but also in any other departments in which privileges may be granted.

Officers of the Medical Staff

The members of the active consulting and the active staffs elect the officers of the medical staff. The officers are accountable to the staff. The officers are the president, the vice-president, and the secretary-treasurer. The elected officers should serve for two years to provide greater stability in working with the rest of the hospital organization. The president and the vice-president are ineligible for reelection.

The president should serve as a member of the medical executive committee but may not serve as the chairperson of the medical executive committee. The president should serve as the presiding officer at all general staff meetings and as the chairperson of the staff advisory council. He or she should represent individual staff members who desire to appeal a decision of the medical executive committee. The president should also have the right to appeal matters to the governing board and to meet with them after discussing a matter with the medical executive committee.

The vice-president or president-elect should serve on the staff advisory council. He or she assumes the presidency when that person's term of office ends. The vice-president may be ineligible for appointment to the medical executive committee.

The secretary-treasurer should be responsible for conducting the balloting for all elected positions of the staff. He or she is also responsible for the disbursement of all staff funds. The secretary-treasurer should be ineligible for appointment to the medical executive committee.

Chapter 10

Performance and Compensation: Evaluating the Board and CEO

Evaluating the performance of a hospital's board of directors and determining whether or not board members should be compensated for their services are relatively new issues in health care governance. Similarly, the best methods for evaluating and compensating CEOs have recently been debated, and many boards are now implementing bonus compensation plans for their chief executives. Because performance and compensation are sensitive issues, they must be raised, discussed, and resolved with great care. Individual performance heavily depends on good working relations, so it is important that the board and the CEO agree on the basis for their evaluation.

Evaluating the Governing Board

Compensation and competence are often intertwined issues. Until a board understands that its performance is crucial to the survival and prosperity of a hospital, it is futile to expect members to consider these matters seriously. Because external forces now affecting hospitals have become so powerful, the experience and wisdom of directors is critical for future survival. The fundamental issue is whether governance is competent to deal with present day operating complexities. Compensation for board service is a secondary matter, useful as a strategy for reinforcing competence.

Basic to examining board effectiveness is the trust relationship between the chairperson of the board and the chief executive. If the chairperson privately believes the chief executive is a poor communicator, has unsatisfactory relations with directors, or is not a mature professional, the process will not work. A suspicion may prevail that the CEO is seeking control of the governing board.

Marketplace and regulatory controls are external forces shaping governing board decisions, particularly since 1983 when Medicare introduced DRGs. Some hospitals prospered during the initial years of the prospective payment system, but nearly all hospitals are now experiencing decreased net surpluses each year. Other concerns have also arisen (see Table 10.1).

These new concerns are complex and require greater competency in the boardroom to deal with them. It is difficult for directors to understand these complexities if they lack an in-depth understanding of the health care industry.

When financial resources were abundant, difficult decisions could be either avoided or delayed until a consensus was achieved. With constrained financial resources, it is no longer possible to approve all proposed capital projects and meet the needs of disenfranchised groups for care.

Poor policy decisions now have long-term effects because future revenues will not be there to offset them. Today, with capped revenues, a major policy decision on a single capital expenditure may well eliminate funding possibilities for other projects. Good board decisions are now critical for future prosperity.

Board characteristics

Policy decisions of a governing board do make a difference. Inept decisions from poorly informed directors risk the future of a hospital. The degree of commitment of board members can be judged by their behavior at board meet-

Table 10.1   Concerns Created by External Forces

Pre-1983	External Force	Concern
High occupancy	Overbedding	Low occupancy
First-dollar coverage	Managed care	Discounted revenues
		Capitated payments
Physician shortage	Physician surplus	Medical staff resistance
No marketing program	Advertising	Market share loss
Physician directed	Carrier driven	HMO/PPO operation
Hospital sharing	Market competition	Hospital wars
Certificate of need	New technology	Outdated technology
Inpatient expansion	Outpatient expansion	Capital shortage

ings. If any of the following characteristics are observable, individual director effectiveness becomes questionable:

- The director never comments adversely or seeks to amend proposed actions and always votes to support recommended policies.
- The director comments after a board meeting that his or her opinions do not matter.
- Agendas are prearranged to sidestep important but controversial decisions.
- The director's approach is always negative and never positive.
- The director is striving to maintain yesterday's reality.

Behavior that demonstrates thoughtfulness, concern, and an understanding of health care issues are characteristics of a competent board of directors.

Important questions for directors

To determine what is important, three questions should be discussed: (1) What programs and accomplishments do directors take greatest pride in? (2) What reputation do directors strive to maintain for the hospital? and (3) Do board members commonly agree on issues or do they often differ substantially on policy decisions?

Substantial differences of opinion between directors indicate a need to reassess the mission statement of a hospital. Board operations and structure may also need to be analyzed. Without common agreement on the goals of a hospital and how they are to be achieved, a board will not be effective.

Sometimes, the initial reaction to board members having differing understandings of a mission is to consider eliminating those directors who disagree. However, it is more useful to examine how the board operates at meetings. A look at the size of a governing board will provide some clues about facilitating or impeding governance functions.

Most directors are sensitive to the feelings and opinions of other members and show respect toward each other in board meetings. They are reluctant to criticize each other because they are voluntarily giving of their time and effort.

The governance processes

Focusing on improving the governance processes avoids individual embarrassment. An outsider is often helpful in such analysis of board operations. An audit of the corporate performance of a board of directors is helpful in examining several factors related to effectiveness. The place to start is a review of board and committee agendas and minutes and observation of board meetings.

Board agendas frequently provide good clues to whether or not major policy issues are avoided or handled in ways that limit discussion. When agendas are arranged with a large number of separate procedural and informational items at the top and major policy matters at the bottom, the discussion of controversial issues will be limited. Reading minutes of board meetings will identify gaming of the agenda.

A second useful method to audit board processes is a review of board minutes of the last three years to count the various types of board activity by categories—procedural, informational, evaluation, policy decisions, and strategic planning. An effective board typically has a high number of evaluation and strategic planning activities.

Observations of board meetings will lead to an understanding of the discussion opportunities provided directors. Such observations reveal the degree to which discussions are consonant with the hospital's mission. If directors are to have a sense that individual participation is important, a board must not be so large that each director does not have enough time to express opinions. Many directors on large boards refrain from speaking on various agenda items to complete an agenda within the scheduled time limits for the meeting.

Review of effectiveness

The chairperson of the board and the chief executive are usually aware of inadequate board performance. The chairperson is usually unwilling to act to improve a board's overall effectiveness unless there are repeated instances of poor behaviors or bad policy decisions. On the other hand, the chief executive may be tempted to take action sooner than the chairperson because bad board decisions create management problems.

When a CEO suggests that the governing board should be evaluated, some directors typically raise questions about ulterior motives. They might think that the CEO wants to reduce the board's authority to increase management's authority. This type of concern can be avoided by having a respected director suggest a board retreat to look at ways to improve board and management effectiveness. Board evaluation should not be a subject for discussion at a regular meeting of the board of directors. A period of uninterrupted time, away from the urgency of daily affairs, is needed for adequate consideration. An outside facilitator is often helpful in getting a board to look at itself and how it is functioning.

CEO concerns

How well a board functions is not only a concern of directors but of vital interest to the CEO. Since most hospital executives do not control the selection of board members, they are unable to directly affect the operations of the board.

When a board meddles in operations, unnecessarily delays approval for projects requiring timely decisions, or rejects worthwhile strategies, a chief executive is handicapped and opportunities are lost. Success in today's health care environment requires innovation and aggressiveness. A CEO needs to be the designer of new strategies but needs the support of the chairperson for success.

Frequently, CEOs privately lament that they could be much more effective if only the board would get out of their way so they could operate the hospital like a corporation. Implicit is the belief that this is the right way to go, even though this belief may be unfounded. A responsible board of directors provides balanced judgments through greater objectivity than can be achieved through an internally driven board. No one individual possesses a comprehensive view and knowledge of all of the external forces affecting health care services. A competent board is not a rubber-stamp for administrative decisions but a necessary screen to ensure adequate consideration and the protection of fundamental values and responsibilities.

A significant criticism of hospital boards is their inability to oversee medical staff activities. When a board waffles on medical staff matters, they are compromising a CEO's effectiveness in the operation of the hospital. Repeated failure of a board to face up to medical staff decisions decreases a chief executive's willingness to trust board decisions. Mistrust often leads to the withholding of information by the CEO and less than total honesty in reporting matters to the board. To a substantial extent, the effectiveness of a board can be determined by its relationship with the CEO. The views of the chief executive on the role and operation of a board are needed to encourage a workable and effective relationship with the directors.

Effective board practices

A board of directors functions effectively when it follows these practices:

- Sets corporate strategies based on the recommendations of the CEO
- Provides counsel on recommended courses of action
- Maintains a reasonable risk-taking posture
- Carries out responsibilities in a timely fashion
- Allows the administration to manage the organization
- Prevents conflicts of interests from arising
- Remains accountable for the commitment of resources
- Makes effective use of individual board member talents
- Seeks to maintain a good public image
- Regularly evaluates the performance of the CEO

Standards of performance

A governing board's effectiveness can be compromised by the performance of individual directors. Individual director judgment and behavior should demonstrate these characteristics:

- A breadth of understanding about health care
- Reasoned judgments on corporate matters
- Acceptance of responsibility
- Concern for carrying out the mission of the hospital
- Maintaining the confidentiality of deliberations
- Adequate preparation for meetings
- Good financial judgment
- An awareness of the board's accountability for the operation of the hospital

An awareness of problems and a willingness to discuss them creates a climate for improved board effectiveness. The appendix at the end of this book provides sample instruments for assessing knowledge gaps that may become the focus of efforts to renew the board and to improve their knowledge.

The process of accomplishing change is unique to each board of directors. The more objective the process, the greater will be its acceptance. Establishing performance standards for board members and an annual individual evaluation can assist in easing a transition to improved effectiveness.

Compensation for service

In developing an evaluation process for measuring board effectiveness, it is useful to discuss the question of compensating directors for their services. However, evaluation might be only a smoke screen for establishing compensation for service on the board.

In the past, hospital boards were typically called boards of trustees. The term originated among charitable organizations sponsored by religious groups. As hospitals broadened their scope of services, they eventually became organized as corporate entities that had charitable missions and were exempt from taxation.

The need to change the trustee ethic

The trustee ethic is pervasive in American society. To become a trustee of a hospital is to feel good about one's self and to fulfill a need to serve others. To accept compensation for such service is to depreciate one's feelings of worthwhileness. Why then, should compensation for service as a trustee be considered? When a hospital board of directors believes that the basic purpose of governance is the well-being of the hospital, compensation should be considered. It is a strategy for encouraging competence at the governance level.

Board effectiveness has two dimensions: the overall corporate functions of governance and the individual performance of directors. Improvement in either dimension increases effectiveness; improvement in both maximizes effectiveness.

Among business corporations, compensation recognizes the director's leadership role by emphasizing the importance of the responsibilities of that body. Paying for services encourages a feeling that the compensation should be earned by personal effort. From management's perspective, there is a feeling that the sense of worth is increased since all elements of the organization are paid for their efforts.

The question of the cost of compensating board members is likely to be raised. When a board is too big, the cost can become a stimulant for decreasing the number of directors. The combined effect of a smaller board coupled with an evaluation process creates a stronger board with improved individual effectiveness.

When struggling with a particularly contentious problem requiring an unusual time commitment, board members sometimes wonder if their efforts are appreciated. If compensation is based on attendance at committee and board meetings, the hospital's appreciation for a director's service becomes directly related to board responsibilities.

Compensation justifies the performance evaluation of individual directors and provides an acceptable reason for not reappointing ineffective board members. Performance evaluations stress individual accountability for board behavior and performance.

Some may argue that individual and corporate effectiveness can be achieved without compensation. Before reaching this conclusion, however, a realistic appraisal of board performance should clearly demonstrate that that is the case.

Problems with compensation

Compensation is not a one-way street. In a few states, paying directors abrogates a liability exemption for directors of not-for-profit hospitals. Losing this protection may reduce the number of desirable director candidates. However, increased accountability for governance is desirable if the result is improved effectiveness.

Director compensation may trigger a medical staff request for payment for their administrative duties, commonly a voluntary activity. Some physicians regularly undertake time-consuming and difficult leadership tasks without seeking compensation even through these duties reduce practice income.

Several large community hospitals have already established payment systems for chiefs of services and also pay members who chair major medical staff committees. Payment for administrative duties for hospital-based medical specialties have been included in the Medicare program since its inception. Payment for these services is justifiable and will undoubtedly become widespread in the future.

How much pay?

The selection of a method of compensation and the rate of pay needs careful thought. Clearly, director fees should not be excessive, to avoid the allegation of private inurement in a not-for-profit hospital. The Internal Revenue Service simply defines these payments as ones that are reasonable, in keeping with director fees paid board members in other nonprofit organizations such as savings and loan associations.

The purpose of compensation is to motivate excellence in individual directors' performance. Obviously, a hospital cannot pay an amount that equals the value of the services provided by directors. Because the officers of a hospital board have greater responsibilities and are frequently involved on an individual basis with the hospital, an annual honorarium may be considered rather than a per diem director's fee for attendance at meetings.

While measurements of standards of performance and compensation are not traditional, they represent steps that are needed in coping with the competitive environment of health care. Compensation begets competence, but it is not a guarantee of success. Each hospital must decide for itself whether or not individual evaluations of performance and compensation for the services of its directors will enhance board performance.

Measuring worth

The concept of annually reviewing the performance of individual members of a governing board of a nonprofit health care organization is not widely used. Traditionally, board members serving voluntarily without compensation has been the norm. They have given of their time as part of their responsibility as good citizens, wishing to be of service. As such, they perceive evaluation as an affront in determining the worthwhileness of their contribution. True or not, trustees simply assume that giving of one's time is a positive contribution to the welfare of the institution.

Today, the work of a governing board and the decisions they reach are vital to the success of a hospital. The trend toward smaller boards means the impact of each board member is proportionately greater. Conversely, failure to adequately contribute is detrimental to the successful operation of the board. As health care resources become scarcer, due to increasing restrictions on payments, emphasis has shifted to ensuring quality of care. The decade of the 1990s will be noteworthy for the health care field's concern with quality. Not only will patient care activities, and those providing it, be subject to greater scrutiny, but quality at all levels and in all activities will be the hallmark of the decade. Measurements of performance that have previously been in place will take on new meaning and be more substantive. As part of the effort to become more quality oriented, it is appropriate to include appraisals of individual board member performance.

The review process

While board members might be willing to accept performance appraisal as necessary and desirable, the question typically arises who will do it. Clearly, whoever conducts the appraisal has to be knowledgeable about the individual's performance throughout the year. Those in a position to make such judgments are, necessarily, also members of the governing board. As would be anticipated, there is usually a reluctance to judge equals in the hierarchy. This reluctance can be overcome in several ways.

All members of the governing board can be asked to prepare an appraisal on every other board member. These can then be turned in to the chairperson for scoring and subsequent decisions. Another method could be to ask each of the executive committee members to appraise all board members except themselves and to then evaluate the collective results. A third possibility is to use either of these methods but then to turn over the completed appraisals to the nominating committee for decision making. This is appropriate since the nominating committee's role is to determine persons to be recommended for board membership. Intrinsic to this responsibility is an evaluation of individuals as part of their annual recommendations.

Following a standard procedure will assist in the individual appraisal. Exhibit 10.1 is an example of an appraisal form that can provide for evaluating board members.

Compensating Chief Executives

With increasing frequency, governing boards are recognizing the desirability of bonus compensation for their chief executives. Once the board decides to provide a bonus, the question arises what basis to use and how much to pay. Governing boards do not like to pick a number out of the air and prefer an objective method for making these bonus decisions.

Several steps are required. The first is a comprehensive employment contract covering both additional compensation and severance. Since a bonus program is retrospective and rewards superior performance, it should focus on overall hospital issues and not only on year-end net profits. Because of the restrictive payment policies of the federal government in its Medicare and Medicaid programs, year-end profits are no longer satisfactory indicators of overall performance. That is not to say that the achievement of approved operating budgets and capital needs should not be used in evaluating performance.

The primary tool for evaluating CEO performance should be the strategic plan that the governing board has adopted. Objectives in the strategic plan and other global matters should be considered as individual criteria for rating performance. A program for determining a bonus should include the following elements.

First, the CEO should have a comprehensive employment contract that includes both a bonus compensation agreement and a reasonable severance arrangement. Severance compensation should ensure personal financial protection for the CEO, against the risks taken for innovative leadership, while also rewarding years of successful service. A minimum of one year's salary and benefits plus one month's salary and benefits for every full year of service, over ten years, are recommended as severance compensation. The employment contract should allow either the board or the CEO to invoke the severance agreement, if the board makes decisions that effectively diminish the CEO's ability to manage the organization.

Second, the strategic plan for the hospital should form the basis of the incentive compensation program. It should be an integral part of the CEO's evaluation. An incentive compensation program tied to the strategic plan will motivate a CEO to produce a realistic plan and improve the implementation of the plan. Each objective should have measurable criteria. An incentive compensation plan should motivate the CEO to focus on both the short- and long-term objectives of the organization.

Third, a bonus program should be retrospective and focus on global issues confronting the hospital. A bonus program relates to the performance evaluation by financially rewarding a CEO for overall positive performance. The amount of the bonus should be calculated as the percent of the CEO's base salary (see Exhibit 10.2).

Fourth, the board of directors needs to adopt a written methodology to use in the evaluation of the CEO that includes a fair evaluation of both objective and subjective information. The CEO should be evaluated against previously established objectives (see Exhibit 10.3). The executive committee should conduct the formal evaluation process, but committee members may seek input from other board members. The executive committee and the CEO should jointly agree on the objectives that form the basis for the CEO's performance evaluation. The CEO should be given one of the following ratings for each objective:

1. Clearly failed to meet the objective
2. Made minimal progress toward the objective
3. Made substantial progress but has not yet completed the objective
4. Completed the objective
5. Exceptional, clearly exceeded the anticipated results of the objective

Exhibit 10.1   Board Member Annual Performance
Appraisal

Name of board member _____

Appraiser _____

Date _____

	Limited	Acceptable	Expected	Impressive	Exemplary
	1	2	3	4	5

1. Commitment
   a. Prepares for meetings
   b. Hospital interests are a high priority
   c. Informed through reading and
      participation in educational programs

2. Understands role
   a. Knows appropriate organizational
      channels of operation
   b. Considers other viewpoints
   c. Accepts consensus versus
      individual position

3. Decision making
   a. Strives to have necessary information
   b. Willing to make decisions with less
      than total information when necessary
   c. Takes appropriate risks
   d. Supports board decisions
   e. Challenges decisions, with cause

4. Analytical skills
   a. States issues and problems clearly
      and concisely
   b. Conclusions reflect good judgment
      and thoughtful evaluation
   c. Understands results of decisions

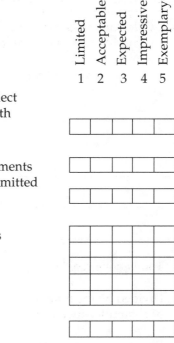

	Limited 1	Acceptable 2	Expected 3	Impressive 4	Exemplary 5

d. Opinions and comments reflect adequate knowledge of health care industry

5. Dependability
   a. Follows through on commitments
   b. Reports and projects are submitted on time

6. Personal traits
   a. Remains poised under stress
   b. Tactful
   c. Appropriate appearance
   d. Gets along with people
   e. Sensitive to other's feelings

Total

Grand total

_____ 22–44   Limited
_____ 45–66   Acceptable
_____ 67–88   Expected
_____ 89–110   Impressive
_____ 111–120   Exemplary

Check appropriate level

Action taken: _____

_____

_____

Reviewed by: _____
                              Signature

Exhibit 10.2   Calculation of Executive Bonus

---

1. Calculate an average committee score from the individual committee member evaluation scores.

Committee Member	*Average Evaluation Score*
_____	_____
_____	_____
_____	_____
_____	_____
_____	_____

Total above scores   _____

Divided by the number
of committee members   _____

Equals the average committee score   _____

2. To calculate the dollar amount of the bonus, use the following chart and equation.

Average Evaluation Score	*Percent of Base Salary*
<2.0	0%
2.0–2.9	5.0%
3.0–3.9	10.0%
4.0–4.4	15.0%
>4.5	20.0%

_____ %   × $_____   = $_____
Percent of   Base salary   Bonus
base salary

Exhibit 10.3   Chief Executive Performance Evaluation

Objectives	(Circle One)				
1. Strategic plan up to date	1	2	3	4	5
2. Capital expenditure budget developed and met	1	2	3	4	5
3. Hospital operating budgets developed and met	1	2	3	4	5
4. Maintains budgeted staffing levels in each department	1	2	3	4	5
5. Maintains compliance with all regulatory agencies	1	2	3	4	5
6. Maintains visible presence within the hospital	1	2	3	4	5
7. Has positive relationships with medical staff leaders	1	2	3	4	5
8. Identifies and evaluates new business opportunities	1	2	3	4	5
9. Remodeling, renovation, and construction project schedules are met	1	2	3	4	5
10. Assists medical staff in physician recruitment	1	2	3	4	5
11. Initiates with the board chairperson and develops board education program	1	2	3	4	5
12. Works toward fellowship status in the American College of Healthcare Executives	1	2	3	4	5

————————— ÷ 12 = —————————

Total points earned   Average evaluation score

Chapter 11

Reforming Health Care Policy:
A Proposal for Change

Having examined the interrelationships between public policy and its impact on hospitals, we have assessed a variety of internal organizational problems created by the ever-changing dynamics involved. This has led to suggesting ways in which a hospital could more effectively cope with this external environment by shoring up important hospital relationships.

Inevitably, thoughtful students of the health care scene must ask themselves if shoring up is all that is required. If present trends in paying hospitals and physicians continue on their course, the answer is apparent: the suggestions fall far short of what is needed. Present trends need to be modified. Those knowledgeable about health care need to be heard, along with other concerned groups. Board members may find a revised national health policy that they can support.

This discussion presents a rationale for revising existing national health care policy and for adopting a new conceptual model that moderates the health care responsibilities of the federal government. There are five parts: the first is an overview of the major forces affecting the national economy in general and health care in particular. Following this, the roles and responsibilities of the health care providers are examined insofar as they are threatened by efforts to reduce the federal deficit. Federal health care policies are then analyzed in terms of congressional patterns, making explicit the implicit assumptions that appear to have been the basis for legislative actions. This leads to an examination of the problems such policies have for providers and the resulting consequences on hospitals.

Because the current federal health care trend is inherently contradictory, a continuation of it without significant revisions will lead to one of two untenable outcomes: a significant and rapid increase in health care funding or a bankrupt health care delivery system requiring significant federal intervention.

Background

In the history of the federal government's involvement in health care, two distinct phases clearly stand out. From the time of the formation of the U.S. Public Health Service in 1798 until 1963, the federal role was limited to public health and to providing direct care for the military, their beneficiaries, and the veterans who served in the armed forces. With the passage of Title XVIII and Title XIX of the Social Security Act (Medicare and Medicaid), the federal government's role dramatically changed to paying for the care of an age-defined segment of the population and another segment that was economically disadvantaged.

When the federal government instituted these programs in 1963, the beneficiaries received units of service, not dollars of care. Dollars were applied only to the units of service to determine the amount that had to be paid to health care providers for the cost of providing services. There were two built-in difficulties. As the cost per unit of service increased, the amount of federal dollars had to increase; and as the units of service provided exceeded the budgeted units of service, still more dollars were needed.

As costs increased per unit of service and the number of units of service exceeded budgeted demand, total cost rose steadily year after year. To slow the rise, DRGs were adopted as a method of payment in 1983. This method paid a lump sum to the hospital for total services rendered per diagnosis to a patient, rather than per unit of service. It is the method currently in use for Medicare and is still widely supported by federal legislators. A number of major factors lie behind congressional support. These include

- deep concern over the growing federal deficit with its gradually increasing interest charges,
- persistent trade imbalances due to global competition with U.S. products,
- public sentiment against tax increases,
- a growing need to increase spending on the national infrastructure,
- a need to prevent an inflationary spiral, and
- the expansion or modification of social programs and entitlements to keep them budget neutral.

These factors, in turn, have profound impacts on the funding of health care by the federal government.

The Impact of Forces Affecting Health Care

Within the health care field, there are a number of trends over which hospitals have no control. These include the following:

- Growing numbers of aged persons entering the Medicare program
- Rapid increase in the number of AIDS patients
- Advances in medical technology requiring large capital expenditures

- Growing surplus of physicians, which continue to be maldistributed
- A shortage of registered nurses
- A shortage of ancillary personnel
- Medicare payments, that pay 44 percent of all patient days of care in hospitals but do not keep pace with inflation
- Federal definitions of Medicare fraud and abuse that interfere with sound marketing strategies
- The application of antitrust laws based on an inappropriate understanding of the nature of health care

As the costs of the Medicare program continue to rise, the federal government has increasingly restricted payments to providers. At the same time, beneficiaries have increasingly been required to pay modest coinsurance and deductible amounts. This approach was the same one the Blue Cross plans followed beginning in the 1950s when they learned that charging a standard premium rate for everybody enrolled (community rating) simply was not workable. This led the Blue Cross plans to experience-rate employee groups. Through the years, hospitals were usually reimbursed for their operating costs, not on a charge for each service provided. During the same period, Blue Shield plans were paying physicians under the usual, reasonable, and customary method of payment.

As Blue Cross operating margins fell, their guiding philosophy of social equity gradually shifted to a concern for financial viability, recognizing that this reality had to be met before social concerns could be considered. By defining units of service rather than dollar protection for Blue Cross, an episode of illness was unhooked from economic consequences since employers paid for employee health insurance. Ultimately, it was recognized that the judicious use of health services required patients to share some degree of economic responsibility for their illness. However, when the federal government adopted the DRG program for Medicare, it placed the economic consequences on the hospital rather than patients. Patients bear a minor economic burden in terms of coinsurance and deductible features. The onus is on the hospital, which cannot bill a patient for hospital costs incurred in their treatment that exceed the payment from Medicare. To hide the inadequacy of funding, government spokespersons have claimed that hospitals are inefficient and mismanaged. This allegation avoids the real issue that the federal government has never lived up to its enacted legislation for hospital payments but has always funded less than called for in the passage of the enabling legislation.

The collective impact of these forces now threatens specific traditional roles and responsibilities of health care providers. Especially endangered are

- the survival of inner city hospitals, which predominantly serve the poor and the needy;
- the survival of acute care general hospitals in rural areas;
- the need for teaching hospitals to continue postgraduate medical education programs;
- ways to increase the supply of registered nurses and ancillary personnel;
- funding for capital costs, to keep up to date on advances in medical technology;
- ways to avoid deterioration in the quality of care as a result of inadequate revenues;
- ways to compete with physicians who offer ambulatory services that duplicate traditional hospital services;
- ways to cope effectively with managed care plans that demand deeper and deeper discounts from providers; and

- support for public hospitals, which provide services for indigent patients.

The prospective payment system Medicare now uses pays a standardized amount per diagnosis. Each diagnostic classification is assumed to pay the hospital for each admission based on a national average case cost. However, the federal government has tilted the tables in its favor by not paying for care beyond the median until the median length of stay exceeds two standard deviations. In practical terms, the hospital pays for all the costs of care beyond the median until the median length of stay has nearly doubled. Beyond that point, the government pays for only 60 percent of the additional amount, and the hospital writes off the remainder. As a result, both the median length of stay and the median cost that were used to establish the DRG system are nonfunctional. Because of the formulas used, hospitals have come to regard the average length of stay as the maximum length of stay.

Patients in need of additional care may be kept beyond the median length of stay if the attending physician believes it is unsafe to discharge them. Like patients, physicians are not economically affected by holding patients beyond the median length of stay. Whenever this occurs, they are only subject to review by the utilization review committee of the hospital. Physicians typically exercise a degree of clinical judgment that is a built-in safety value for the Medicare program and works to the advantage of the federal payment system. If the physician deems it advisable to keep the patient beyond the median length of stay, the cost is borne by the hospital, not the federal program.

This federal practice is based on the tradition that not-for-profit hospitals are social agencies and ignores the changes that have taken place. Not-for-profit hospitals are now major employers in their communities and are substantial business enterprises. Hospitals must now give equal weight to the financial issues and their social concerns as hospital revenues become further constrained. Hospital efforts are further hampered by congressional decision making that has failed to recognize the competitive marketplace in which they now operate.

Congressional Patterns

Up to now, national health care policy has been developed on an incremental basis. As a result, it is implicit, inconsistent, and contradictory. Under the prospective payment system, this piecemeal pattern of policy making directly threatens the survival of health care providers. Table 11.1 illustrates the pattern of implicit congressional policies and the problems the providers face as a consequence of these decisions.

Contradictions between Regulation and Marketplace Realities

Beyond the pressures now facing providers as a consequence of past policies, a myriad of regulatory restrictions apply to health care. Providers are prohibited from applying sound marketing principles to thwart competitive threats to their institutional survival. Several examples are cited in Table 11.2.

Outcomes

Congress's philosophy appears to be to continue the existing Medicare and Medicaid programs but, at the same time, to restrict payments to providers. The inescapable conclusion is that it simply cannot work. Two outcomes can be foreseen:

1. If equal health care benefits are provided to all citizens, the federal government must rapidly and

Table 11.1 Congressional Patterns

Implicit or Explicit Policy	Providers' Problems	Consequences to Providers
Access for all	Inadequate financing	Mission or margin Irrational hospital closures
Coverage for uninsured	Closing emergency rooms Increasing bad debts	Providers at risk
Coverage for underinsured	Employers move employees from full-time to part-time	No coverage to pay bills
The expansion of Medicare to nonacute care (drugs, etc.)	Recipients don't understand coverage limits and blame hospitals	Contractual adjustments increase at a faster rate
Acceptable quality of care to all citizens	Lack of definition of quality of care	Increase in law suits
Part B payments are out of control and need to be controlled	Increase in number of physicians refusing to care for Medicare patients	Limits access
Increasing Medicare enrollment funded out of existing funds	Developing greater productivity Finding offsetting sources of revenue Restricting salary increases to employees	Increase in transfers to public hospitals Other carriers refuse to permit cost-shifting Loss of personnel

Table 11.2   Regulators' versus Hospitals' Viewpoints on
Health Care Issues

Regulators' Viewpoint	*Hospitals' Viewpoint*
1. Fraud and abuse regulations protect the patient and the federal government.	1. They interfere with the extent and variety of incentives for higher productivity.
2. Certificates of need control unnecessary building programs.	2. a. They interfere with sound economic and social programming. b. They restrict a hospital's ability to compete with other health care providers.
3. Antitrust rules economically protect the patient from financial abuse.	3. Antitrust rules increase the cost of health care.
4. Rate regulation protects the public in four states.	4. Rate regulation interferes with keeping up to date in technology.
5. Incremental increases in programs can be financed piecemeal or hidden in existing funding.	5. Programming has to be explicitly tied to specific funding.
6. Medicare expenditures have been increasing 11 percent and must be constrained.	6. a. Medicare outlays should increase to accommodate additional enrollees. b. Absence of inflation adjustments in Medicare payments threatens to bankrupt hospitals.
7. The primary concern is meeting one-year budget goals.	7. Long-term survival is the primary concern.

substantially increase expenditures for health care. If existing Medicare benefits are increased, the financing for these benefits must come from sources other than increased efficiency in hospital operations.

2. If federal funding for health care cannot be increased, or is decreased, one of the following scenarios will ensue:

   a. The federal government will redefine its responsibilities in health care and adopt a more modest role in keeping with its ability to finance the commitments it makes.

   b. The legitimate financial interests of hospitals will go unrecognized until there are significant institutional bankruptcies and patient care is being denied to federally sponsored individuals. To prevent a major collapse of the hospital system, a national health care system may be legislated, adopting a strong, centrally controlled authority that has responsibility for balancing revenues and expenditures.

A National Health Care System

A national health care system may offer several advantages to the federal government:

1. Existing dynamics and rapid change affecting health care funding could be blunted through central control and authority.

2. A central authority could determine needs and allocate resources through various parts of the system.

3. The level of expenditures for health care could be harmonized with the availability of funds.

4. Federal health care expenditures could be kept in balance with other elements of the federal budget.

Assuming that a national health care service is desirable and covers all the costs of illness for the total population, the question arises how much it would cost. Several years ago, John R. Mannix, formerly the president of the Cleveland Blue Cross Plan, analyzed this question and determined that, at that time, the individual federal income tax would have to be increased by 90.1 percent, based on the existing utilization patterns of all the existing health care services. On balance, it seems likely that in spite of anticipated corporate and governmental pressures for a national health care program, the tax increase required to fund it would meet with considerable opposition from the general public.

The Alternative

Under existing strategies, the federal government has only one avenue in dealing with hospitals. It must restrict the level of payments to providers because it has no control over the number of units of service either hospitals or physicians provide. Since the federal government has no direct responsibility for providing patient care, it is likely to continue to respond to the needs of the federal budget more than the funding needs of hospitals. This annual funding shortfall will greatly increase mandated benefits. Should the point be reached where physicians and hospitals withdraw from the Medicare program, the ability of the government to live up to its commitments would be jeopardized. To avoid having to face the prospect of a national health insurance program, congressional philosophy on health care should be redefined.

Two questions need to be answered for an alternative philosophy: (1) What is the appropriate role for the federal government, in keeping with its limited ability to fund health care? (2) What steps can the federal government take to encourage a free market to respond to health care needs not funded by the federal government? Table 11.3 responds to these issues.

Table 11.3   Conceptual Framework for a National Health Care Philosophy

	Benefits	Financing Mechanism	Eligibility	Providers
Mandated	Catastrophic coverage	SSA (individual contributions)	Mandated for employed persons Voluntary enrollment	Acute care hospitals Physicians
Free market	Elective coverage	Third party payers Commercial Blue Cross HMO PPO Self-pay	Determined by coverage	Free choice or determined by coverage
Mandated minimum standards	Mandated minimum coverage	Voucher Government purchase Free market purchase	Third party payers licensed	Free choice or determined by coverage

If the dynamic changes occurring in the health care field continue, it will be necessary to avoid a centralized control that (1) locks the status quo into place, (2) greatly inhibits organizational modifications, (3) prevents shifts in the use of resources, and (4) lessens efforts to advance medical technology. At the same time, it is also unreasonable to leave health care in the hands of an unrestricted free marketplace. A mix of government and the free market is needed. Certain principles need to be agreed on.

Principles

If a combination of government and a free marketplace are used to develop a stable program, the following principles need to be recognized:

1. Health care is best provided when it is responsive to the local level and requires decisions to be made at that level. Two basic factors drive the local nature of health care:
   a. Sick people seek the emotional support of family members. When they are hospitalized, they prefer a local hospital, to have the support of their families.
   b. Primary care physicians much prefer to use local medical consultants or to refer to other local physicians because referrals are informal and highly subjective.
2. The federal government's responsibility is to establish a ceiling of health care costs beyond which a national catastrophic coverage program should assume the costs.
3. For those who cannot obtain coverage, the federal government should provide a voucher that can be used to purchase coverage for basic benefits from a provider.

4. The free market should operate below the level of catastrophic care except for those categories of disadvantaged citizens who are provided vouchers.

Maximum and Minimum Levels

The basic building block for a national health care policy is that patients are entitled to avoid bankruptcy from an illness, either acute or chronic. Eligibility for participation must be open to all individuals—nonworking individuals, students, employees, and retirees—all persons in the country regardless of their social or financial well-being.

A second need is to determine the minimum level of coverage for every citizen. For those organizations that want to compete in the free marketplace, there should be a certification to ensure they offer benefits equal or superior to the established minimum standards. For the disadvantaged and those unable to pay, the government (preferably at the federal level) should issue a voucher that can be used to purchase minimum coverage in a person's local area.

Catastrophic Coverage Principles

In planning for catastrophic coverage the basic principles should be

1. to cover as many persons as possible in the program so that a normal distribution curve is approximated,
2. to commence coverage at a high enough dollar level that the monthly premium cost is modest,
3. to provide coverage only for acute care in hospitals but to pay all associated hospital costs and professional fees, and
4. to provide a simple way of paying premiums for the coverage.

Obtaining a normal distribution curve

Catastrophic coverage should be designed for the general public and not for a segment of the population. From a statistical standpoint, the worst possible choice to use for determining catastrophic coverage is the 65 and over population, the Medicare enrollees. This segment uses the greatest amount of hospital resources, at a rate five times that of persons under age 65.

The best choice is to provide coverage to all age groups in the population. To ensure a normally distributed curve of health care costs, the program must be mandatory.

Catastrophic coverage should be available to Medicare enrollees as well as to all other groups, including

1. a growing number of employees shifted from full-time to part-time employment by employers to avoid paying fringe benefits;
2. ex-spouses who had coverage in a group plan when they were married but are unable to secure individual coverage after divorce because of a preexisting condition;
3. emancipated minors attending universities who totally rely on student health care services because they cannot afford individual coverage;
4. persons who have group coverage when working for a corporation but, when they leave it to start a small business, cannot afford to buy insurance as an individual or cannot obtain it because of a preexisting condition; and
5. persons who do not qualify for Medicaid because they earn too much but cannot afford to purchase health insurance.

Two issues need to be carefully explored before catastrophic coverage is provided across the board for all illnesses: (1) the monthly premium level that can be charged that permits the enrollment of the entire population and (2) the threshold level (in dollars) for catastrophic coverage when it includes acute care, nursing home care, outpatient care, rehabilitation, and psychiatric services.

Coverage level

The purpose of catastrophic coverage is to limit the amount of money an individual or his or her primary insurance company is to pay for hospital care. The objective in establishing a threshold for catastrophic coverage is to set the base at a point where only a small percentage of patients will qualify. The higher the percentage of patients that reach the threshold, the higher the monthly premium must be. It might be desirable in the early years of catastrophic coverage to give priority to the monthly premium cost and set the coverage accordingly, rather than the reverse. The primary question is how much an individual or an employer is willing to pay to have a known dollar level beyond which there are no additional costs for hospitalization.

To keep the monthly premium modest, the focus should be on how much coverage can be bought at a specific premium level. If the focus is allowed to shift to the comprehensiveness of care and coverage is broadened to such services as nursing homes, prescription drugs, and other health services, the monthly premium will begin to rise, with the risk that increasing portions of the population will become dissatisfied. Should the premium rate be held low but benefits gradually expanded to a wider range of services, the government may once again find itself paying for more health care than budgetary constraints allow.

Extent of coverage

A main advantage of a national catastrophic coverage program is to permit a free market to operate below the threshold level for catastrophic coverage. Commercial insurance, HMOs, Blue Cross, PPOs, Medicare, and Medicaid should be allowed to continue to compete and provide coverage.

Insurance should initially be limited to acute hospital care and the associated professional fees, until utilization data are sufficiently refined to permit the development of a sound actuarial basis for determining premiums. No comparable data currently exist for nursing homes, rehabilitation programs, psychiatric institutions, home health care programs, or prescription drugs.

The need for a sound data base in catastrophic coverage is so important that only acute care but not extended coverage should initially be considered. No one really knows how much nursing home care might be used if it is available through catastrophic coverage. To include other elements of care without knowing their use rates would defeat the purpose of the program. Demonstration projects in selected areas should be undertaken for each additional program to develop a reliable data base for actuarial purposes.

Paying for catastrophic care

For a national program to be successful, the monthly premium should meet two criteria: (1) a modest cost acceptable to all segments of the population and (2) an easy method of payment.

The Social Security Administration offers the best avenue to explore. Monthly payments could be made using the existing rules so that part-time and full-time employees would be covered. Like FICA, it would be mandatory for the employed population. Coverage should also be available to self-employed persons as well as the unemployed who wish to participate as individuals and thus be obtainable by the entire population. Local and state governments should also be eligible to make contributions for Medicaid recipients, which would make these patients more financially acceptable to health care providers.

A method of payment for hospital providers would need to be determined. Past experience indicates that cost reimbursement is unsatisfactory as a method of payment. Equally unsatisfactory is the DRG method because of the abuses the HCFA has initiated. Though time consuming, the most satisfactory solution might be an annual negotiated rate between the HCFA, or its intermediaries, and individual hospitals. In some communities it might be desirable to bid competitively for catastrophic patients. If so, patients would be transferred to contract hospitals when catastrophic coverage commences. In most instances, such a transfer is safe since the patient's condition is stable and the primary concerns are the economics of the medical care.

To provide catastrophic-level care, there should be as little disruption as possible in the continuum of patient care. To avoid transferring patients, it might be more desirable to not require a transfer to another facility simply to satisfy the financing mechanism. If the federal role is limited to a financial one, an alternative would be to have the provider charge the catastrophic fund only the lowest contract rate it has with a commercial carrier. Retrospective audits make this approach relatively easy to monitor. It also has the advantage of not having the federal government determine rates by geographic areas or rural versus urban differences. In effect, rates would be set by the marketplace conditions in each community. The federal government would simply take advantage of the lowest available rate.

Since contract rates are subject to change, the federal program would need to require that the individual catastrophic contract with a provider remain in place for one year before being subject to change.

Conflicting Federal Policies

When attempting to define a federal health care policy for a minimum level of coverage, the issue becomes more difficult. On the one hand there is a desire to continue an exemption from taxation for health care benefits, which is now unequal for taxpayers because the dollar amounts employees pay for health care premiums vary and result in a tax inequity. Employees who have extensive benefits as part of employment are treated (tax-wise) the same as employees who participate in programs that provide minimal benefits. The congressional conflict arises over the question whether health care benefits are primarily a tax matter or primarily a health care matter. Treated as a tax, there is inequity, but viewed from a perspective of health care policy, the more comprehensive the protection, the better it is from a social perspective.

Another concern is the need to provide health care coverage for the 38 million persons who are uninsured. If Congress determines that the uninsured are a responsibility of the federal government, then two questions must be answered about who pays for coverage and what is the extent of coverage. If traditional methods were used, tax dollars would be allocated and first-day coverage would be provided. The dilemma then becomes whether to further unbalance the federal budget for the additional people covered or to seek an alternative that places the financing responsibility elsewhere. It might be worthwhile to initiate a voucher system for purchasing a basic benefits package in the local community.

The Other Side of the Coin

After looking at the catastrophic benefit, the next step is to look at the minimum benefits every citizen should have for acute care. Assuming that the federal government adopts such a position, additional questions need to be answered: (1) How extensive should minimum benefits be? (2) How should a minimum benefit program be audited to ensure that all citizens participate? (3) What sources of funding should be used?

To determine the extent of minimum benefits is a difficult problem in terms of the type of health care. There already are a wide variety of programs offering coverage, including those sponsored by the federal government (e.g., Medicare, Medicaid, and the Civilian Health and Medical Program of the Uniformed Services [CHAMPUS]) and those sponsored by for-profit and not-for-profit organizations such as Blue Cross/Blue Shield and other commercial carriers in the private sector. Should all of these programs be permitted to stay in place as long as they meet the minimum standards of coverage? Existing benefits under each plan could be converted to dollars of coverage similar to indemnity coverages.

The minimum benefit level is quite different from the problem of the level of catastrophic coverage. The development of a catastrophic program would fill a gap largely missing today. As a result, there is little concern that it would duplicate existing coverages, which allows a plan to be implemented with relative ease and minimal disruption of existing coverages.

Application of a Deductible

While deductibles and coinsurance do not deter hospitalization, these insurance features do affect the number of visits to a physician office. By placing a deductible between the patient and visits to the physician's office, use of the health care system is deterred. Deterrence can become even more effective if the deductible is applied monthly rather than annually.

In computing such a deductible, the following formula might be considered:

$$\frac{\text{Annual employer and employee Social Security contributions for an individual}}{12 \text{ months}} \times \frac{\text{Percent of GDP for}}{\text{health care}}$$

Two examples illustrate this method:

Example 1

1. The individual's annual income is the maximum used under Social Security—$60,600.
2. The employer and employee combined contribution is 15.3 percent of annual income—$9,272.
3. Divide the combined contribution by 12—$773.
4. Multiply that by health care spending of 13.4 percent of the GDP—$103.58.
5. The monthly deductible is $103.58, or $1,242.98 for the year.

Example 2

1. The individual's annual income is $20,000.
2. The employer and employee combined contribution at 15.3 percent is $3,060.
3. Divided by 12 is $255.
4. Multiplied by 13.4 percent for health care spending as a percentage of the GDP is $34.17.
5. The monthly deductible is $34.17, or $410 for the year.

Standardizing the deductible through the use of a formula assures fairness, but at the same time, the deductible amount will vary from year to year since it is based on the combined Social Security contribution and the health care component of the GDP.

The application of this type of deductible could be either mandatory or optional for carriers, whether government or private industry. If it is optional, each financing mechanism would be free to make such a determination. For example, CHAMPUS and Medicare might elect to continue existing benefits unchanged, while some of the Blue

Cross and Blue Shield programs and commercial carriers might elect to apply it. On the other hand, making a legislated deductible mandatory has the following advantages:

- The playing field is level for all persons.
- It clearly communicates a national policy linking the use of the health care system with economic consequences.
- It standardizes the deductible for carriers.
- For the disadvantaged, the voucher would not only facilitate enrollment of individuals in a local plan at the basic benefits level but would eliminate the requirement for coinsurance.

Conclusions

The aim of this proposal is not to address all the fiscal considerations of a health care system. Rather, it is to provide maximum financial support to those few patients who face financial disaster from illness and eliminate a statement that only Americans can make: This is the only country where you can go broke from illness if you don't have the right kind of health insurance. At the minimum benefits level and up to the catastrophic level, it is designed for the operation of a free market while at the same time providing a method for covering the uninsured.

The characteristics of the health care industry are changing. What was true yesterday is no longer true today and will change again tomorrow. These changes make it difficult to develop and maintain a health care policy that serves the public interests in the foreseeable future, yet a new federal policy is urgently needed. If it is to be successful, it must fit within the budgetary constraints of the federal government. This will require a clear sense of priorities for the health care needs of the public. Attempting to an-

swer all of these needs with an elegant solution that is all
encompassing will surely lead away from and not toward
the desired result. An incremental, carefully thought out
public policy would seem to be more desirable.

Appendix

Two Instruments for Identifying Ways to Improve Leadership

Because board members, physicians, and hospital executives are years beyond the completion of their formal educations, they learn and gain insights about hospitals through informal experiences. Board members learn when attending board meetings, reading background material, and, once or twice a year, through attendance at a health care seminar. Physicians learn more about hospitals' activities and responsibilities by participating in departmental meetings; as committee members; as clinical chiefs and chairpersons; by serving on the medical executive committee; and perhaps as the president of the medical staff, who attends and participates as a member of the governing board.

While hospital executives typically have greater experience and contact with the organizational aspects of the hospital than do board members or physicians, they also learn through participation in seminars and continuing education programs. In essence, adults learn about hospital organization and its current environment by thinking through the issues at hand. The two questionnaires in this appendix are designed to give board members, physicians, and executives an opportunity to be individually and personally engaged in a learning process that will contribute to effective governance and leadership in their organizations.

Hospital Governance Questionnaire

All organizations operate at two levels: the formal one, as partially defined by written financial statements, bylaws, policy manuals, and position descriptions, and the informal level where matters are handled subjectively and through oral conversations that do not result in written documents or communications. Both are needed and useful in making an organization operate successfully. However, written communications constitute the reference points by which an organization determines where it is headed.

Successful organizations have established ways of controlling and evaluating their leadership. Because hospitals primarily depend on voluntary, part-time, and usually unpaid board members for leadership and medical staff officers typically unfettered by organizational limits, hospitals have not carefully structured ways to do their business.

The Hospital Governance Questionnaire provides an easy and quick way to identify areas of weakness at the apex of the organization and suggests ways to improve the leadership of the hospital by more clearly expressing expectations.

There are no right or wrong responses. The numbered questionnaire statements are meant to identify organizational practices generally considered to be desirable for an effective governing board. The choices provided reflect different methods of carrying out each practice. Some choices are more desirable than others. For example, a review of the CEO's performance can occur annually, from time to time, or informally. Clearly, the ideal is a regular basis, as occurs annually. Local practices will determine the most desirable response.

Hospital Governance Questionnaire

Organizational performance

Yes   No

1. Written position descriptions have been developed for the following:
   a. The chairperson of the governing board   —— ——
   b. Members of the governing board   —— ——
   c. The chairperson of the executive committee of the governing board   —— ——
2. Written guidelines are prepared and used for describing the roles of each board committee.   —— ——
3. The governing board has adopted criteria for the selection of its members.   —— ——
4. The governing board has adopted criteria to be used in evaluating the performance of the CEO.   —— ——

Individual performance

1. The performance of every member of the governing board is appraised
   a. Annually   —— ——
   b. At the end of the term of the appointment   —— ——
   c. Informally   —— ——
   d. By completing an appraisal form   —— ——
2. Reappointment to the governing board is conditioned on the results of performance appraisal.   —— ——

	Yes	No

3. The performance review is conducted by the
   a. Chairperson of the board   _____ _____
   b. Executive committee   _____ _____
   c. Nominating committee   _____ _____
   d. Chief executive   _____ _____

Chief executive performance

1. The chief executive is a voting member of the governing board.   _____ _____
2. The CEO's performance is reviewed
   a. Annually   _____ _____
   b. From time to time   _____ _____
   c. Informally   _____ _____
3. The performance review is conducted by the
   a. Chairperson of the board   _____ _____
   b. Executive committee   _____ _____
   c. Officers of the corporation   _____ _____
   d. Selected board members   _____ _____

Patient care performance

1. Written position descriptions are developed and used for the
   a. Chief of staff or president of the medical staff   _____ _____
   b. Chiefs of services or department chairpersons   _____ _____
   c. Section chiefs   _____ _____

Yes   No

2. The governing board appoints the following positions:

   a. Chiefs of staff or president of the medical staff   _____ _____

   b. Chiefs of services or department chairpersons   _____ _____

   c. Section chiefs   _____ _____

3. The medical executive committee is accountable to the

   a. Governing board   _____ _____

   b. General medical staff   _____ _____

4. The granting of clinical privileges to individual medical staff members is a responsibility of the

   a. Governing board   _____ _____

   b. Medical executive committee   _____ _____

   c. General medical staff   _____ _____

5. The credentialing process for applicants to the medical staff includes

   a. References   _____ _____

   b. Evaluation of prior training and experience   _____ _____

   c. Proctoring of requested privileges for a predetermined number of cases   _____ _____

6. The fundamental purpose of a medical staff organization is to

   a. Protect and assure patient safety or   _____ _____

   b. Protect the interests of staff members   _____ _____

	Yes	No

7. The reappointment of a medical staff
   member and the extent of privileges
   granted is a decision of

   a. The general medical staff   ____ ____

   b. The medical executive committee   ____ ____

   c. A joint conference committee   ____ ____

   d. The governing board   ____ ____

Hospital Query Quotient

Policy directives for an organization require an understanding of the organization's structure, legal responsibilities, governance processes, and financing to be effective. The Hospital Query Quotient (HQ²) was developed to identify key concepts trustees and medical staff leaders need to carry out their responsibilities. It has been used at hospital retreats to demonstrate key health care concepts and to identify misinformation that may adversely affect policy development.

The questionnaire has five sections: legal, medical staff organization, governing board organization, patient care, and general and finance issues. On the answer sheet, the person's position in the organization is recorded—trustee, physician, or administration—to identify individual and group awareness of key concepts. Answers are tabulated for each group to determine the average level of understanding. Physicians and trustees typically average 50 to 55 percent correct responses. The administrative staff usually correctly respond to 75 percent of the items.

Hospital Query Quotient (HQ²)

Legal   Answer

1. In a hospital, who is ultimately legally
   responsible for the quality of medical care?
   a. The governing board
   b. The medical staff
   c. The chief executive
   d. The medical executive committee   _____

2. The hospital is perceived to engage in the
   corporate practice of medicine when
   a. It employs physicians on a salary basis
   b. The chief executive contracts with an
      industrial plant to provide preemployment
      physicals to prospective employees
   c. Emergency room physicians on salary have
      admitting privileges
   d. None of the above   _____

3. When a hospital creates a parent-subsidiary
   type health care corporation, the hospital is
   typically
   a. The parent corporation
   b. A subsidiary
   c. An unrelated party
   d. A management company   _____

4. When a hospital forms a philanthropic foundation, the two are legally unrelated if
   a. The majority of board members of the foun-
      dation are not associated with the hospital
      in an official capacity

Answer

   b. The proceeds of the foundation may be
      given to other health-related organizations
      as well as to the hospital

   c. The foundation meets separately from the
      hospital

   d. Either (a) or (b)   _____

5. A nonprofit hospital jeopardizes its tax-
   exempt status when

   a. The majority of its revenue is derived
      from for-profit activities in other related
      corporations

   b. The bottom line (net surplus) exceeds 20
      percent

   c. The hospital subsidizes the office rent of
      selected physicians

   d. The hospital pays the malpractice premiums
      of the medical staff   _____

Medical Staff Organization

6. Membership on the medical staff of a community voluntary nonprofit hospital is a

   a. Privilege granted by the medical staff

   b. Right inherent by being licensed in the
      state

   c. Privilege granted by the governing board

   d. A decision of the medical executive
      committee   _____

7. Credentials of applicants to the medical staff
   are presented to the governing board as

   a. Required by state law

   b. A matter of courtesy by the medical staff

Answer

   c. A requirement of the hospital

   d. Required by federal law   _____

8. Once medical staff bylaws are approved by the medical staff and forwarded to the governing board, the directors

   a. Must concur

   b. May revise and modify bylaws only with medical staff approval

   c. May rewrite and adopt bylaws over the objections of the medical staff

   d. May approve bylaws only after they have been approved by all clinical departments   _____

9. To establish organizational accountability, a clinical department of the medical staff in a community hospital should

   a. Determine for itself the member of the department who shall be chairperson or chief

   b. Recommend to the governing board the member of the department who should become chairperson or chief

   c. Decide for itself not to have a chairperson or chief

   d. Leave the decision to the governing board   _____

10. The governing board of a hospital can terminate the privileges of any members of the medical staff

   a. At any time, with or without due process

   b. Only if recommended by the medical staff

   c. Only if recommended by the medical executive committee

   d. At any time if it follows its own adopted procedures   _____

Answer

11. The medical executive committee is
    organizationally accountable to
    a. The general medical staff
    b. The administration of the hospital
    c. The governing board
    d. Both the medical staff and governing
       board _____

12. Self-governance of a medical staff is a
    a. Right of the medical staff
    b. Delegation from the governing board
    c. Right conferred by state law
    d. Requirement of the American Medical
       Association _____

13. The governing board assures itself of the
    quality of medical care by
    a. Indicating to the medical staff that they
       should define the process and then im-
       plement the clinical review of cases
    b. Defining the process and then following
       up regularly and continuously to see that
       it is being used
    c. Expecting the CEO to report regularly on
       the clinical activities of the medical staff
    d. Having medical staff representatives on
       the governing board _____

14. If the governing board finds the medical
    staff's clinical review of cases suspect, it has
    the authority to
    a. Seek outside, competent clinical review of
       cases
    b. Ask the medical executive committee to
       tighten up on reviews

Answer

c. Insist that the defined process of clinical review be followed and honestly applied

d. All of the above   _____

15. When a hospital restricts the size and composition of the medical staff, it is not subject to antitrust action if the

a. Entire medical staff indicates and approves the action

b. Governing board and medical staff jointly approve the proposed plan

c. Governing board acts independently

d. Medical executive committee initiates the program   _____

16. When a member of the medical staff requires disciplining, it is the initial responsibility of the

a. Chief of the member's service or section

b. Chief of staff or president

c. CEO of the hospital

d. Medical director   _____

17. The primary purpose of an organized medical staff in a hospital is to

a. Protect the interests of the individual physician

b. Provide management with an organized way of dealing with physicians

c. Provide a mechanism by which the governing board can ensure patient safety through accountability for the quality of medical care

d. Ensure that each physician has a vote on medical staff matters   _____

Answer

18. When a physician on the medical staff becomes a member of the governing board, his or her first responsibility as a member of that body is to

    a. Represent the medical staff to the board
    b. Represent the board to the medical staff and vice versa
    c. Counterbalance the influence of the CEO
    d. Ensure the quality of medical care rendered in the hospital   _____

19. The membership of the medical executive committee should be primarily composed of

    a. Chiefs of service (chairpersons of clinical departments) and at-large members
    b. Members of the medical staff at large, excluding chiefs of service
    c. Hospital-based physicians
    d. Specialists   _____

20. The granting of temporary privileges to a physician should be determined by the

    a. Chiefs of service
    b. Chief executive of the hospital
    c. Chiefs of service in consultation with the chief executive
    d. Chief of staff or president of the staff   _____

21. The CEO or his or her representative attends medical staff committee meetings as a prerogative of

    a. The medical staff
    b. Executive authority
    c. The governing board

Answer

d. The bylaws of the medical staff as approved by the governing board   _____

22. A member of the governing board may attend a committee meeting of the medical staff

    a. Only by the invitation of the medical staff
    b. At the request of the governing board
    c. At the request of the chief executive
    d. Only by the invitation of the chairperson of the committee   _____

23. A medical staff desiring to prevent additional physicians from being accepted as members of that body should

    a. Adopt a resolution of the general medical staff and forward it as a recommendation to the governing board
    b. Adopt resolutions in each clinical department and forward them to the medical executive committee for final approval
    c. Request the governing board and chief executive to investigate the situation and develop a plan if warranted
    d. Informally tell applicants the staff is closed   _____

24. When a hospital employs a full-time medical director, his or her role includes

    a. Establishing and providing oversight on the quality of medical care
    b. Guiding disciplinary interventions with individual medical staff members
    c. Assisting in developing and implementing medical staff policies
    d. All of the above   _____

Governing board organization Answer

25. The primary role of the governing board is to
    a. Regularly review in detail the operations of the hospital
    b. Review all expenditures and approve them
    c. Review and act on the operational and professional policies for guiding the institution
    d. Relate hospital programs to community need _____

26. When a governing board has a number of committees, the typical authority of each committee is to
    a. Make decisions within its authority and to see that they are implemented without reference to the full board
    b. Make recommendations within its charge to the full board
    c. Do both, depending on circumstances
    d. Report only at annual meetings of the corporation _____

27. *Ex officio* means
    a. Participates in discussions by virtue of the office but has no vote
    b. Participates in the discussions with vote, by virtue of the office, unless specifically prohibited by the bylaws
    c. Votes only when asked to do so by the chairperson
    d. Immediate past office holder _____

28. According to Roberts Rules of Order, in the conduct of a board meeting,

Answer

  a. Any board member may introduce a new
     item of business without reference to the
     agenda

  b. A board member must confer with the
     chairperson with regard to an intent to
     introduce new business

  c. The agenda cannot be vacated without a
     majority vote of the governing board on
     the initiation of the chairperson

  d. A board member has to wait until the next
     board meeting to introduce new business   _____

29. When a governing board delegates an activity
    to a subordinate group or person, it should
    delineate

  a. The authority that is authorized and the
     accountability required

  b. The boundaries of the responsibilities
     involved

  c. The measures of accountability required

  d. All of the above   _____

30. The governing board should have the re-
    sponsibility of approving the fee structures
    of the following physicians:

  a. All members of the medical staff

  b. None

  c. Hospital-based specialists under contract
     to the institution

  d. Emergency room physicians only   _____

31. The authority of the chairperson of the
    governing board is

  a. As the chief executive of the hospital

  b. As the presiding officer at meetings of the
     governing board

c. Unabridged

d. As a decision maker between board
   meetings _____

32. When a physician of the medical staff is
    appointed to the governing board, he or she is

    a. At risk for liability, as are other directors
    b. Not subject to conflict of interests require-
       ments
    c. Expected to pass clinical judgments on
       disciplinary actions taken against members
       of the medical staff
    d. To be compensated for his or her services _____

Patient care

33. When experimental drugs or procedures are
    to be used on a patient, the physician should

    a. Seek prior approval from the chief of
       services and inform the patient
    b. Proceed on his or her own after alerting
       the nursing staff of any potential delete-
       rious side effects
    c. Tell the patient what he or she is doing
       and proceed
    d. Seek prior approval from the appropriate
       medical staff committee and inform the
       patient _____

34. Suppose a physician writes an elective order
    on a patient that the nurse believes is not
    good clinical judgment. The nurse communi-
    cates his or her concerns to the physician, but
    the doctor makes no change. The nurse
    should then

    a. Carry out the order as written

Answer

   b. Report the matter to the head nurse after carrying out the order

   c. Immediately report the matter to the head nurse and not carry out the order

   d. Informally report the matter to the chief of service after carrying out the order   _____

35. If an attending physician abuses a patient in the hospital, the initial action should be taken by

   a. The chief of service

   b. The medical executive committee

   c. Leaving the matter to the judgment of the attending physician

   d. The CEO of the hospital   _____

36. If numerous incidents of poor medical judgment occur with respect to an individual member of the medical staff, the

   a. Chief of service should review the matter with the medical executive committee and adopt an appropriate plan of action that the physician is required to follow

   b. Chief of service should review the matter with the medical executive committee and an appropriate plan of action should be adopted that is recommended to the physician but left up to the physician's discretion to decide

   c. Hospital should notify its insurance carrier that it is not involved

   d. Medical executive committee should unilaterally restrict the physician's privileges   _____

Answer

37. When a surgeon decides he or she needs a new surgical instrument to be purchased by the hospital, he or she should
    a. Interview the sales representative and place the order
    b. Request the operating room supervisor to purchase the instrument
    c. Buy it with personal funds and request payment from the hospital
    d. Request the purchasing agent of the hospital to buy the instrument   _____

38. When a physician continues to inappropriately classify his or her patients to secure their admission to the hospital, the
    a. Chief executive should recommend that the governing board suspend his or her admitting privileges
    b. Chief executive should request that the appropriate chief of service to take disciplinary action
    c. Chief executive should request that the appropriate chief of service investigate the matter and then discuss his or her findings with CEO before proceeding any further
    d. Medical executive committee should investigate the situation   _____

General and financial

39. The average tenure of a CEO in community nonprofit hospitals is
    a. Under 2 years
    b. 2–5 years

Answer

c. 6–10 years

d. 11 years or more   _____

40. Traditional hospital corporate structures are giving way to innovative multiple corporate organizations. The reason behind this movement is

   a. To minimize the control of operations by regulatory agencies

   b. To maximize income from health-related enterprises

   c. To protect the market share of the hospital

   d. All of the above   _____

41. Which factor most affects the ability of a hospital to acquire long-term debt?

   a. Mix of reimbursement

   b. High occupancy

   c. Low operating costs

   d. Overall historical financial performance   _____

42. Total operating revenues are defined as

   a. Total operating revenue minus bad debts

   b. Total operating revenues minus charity work

   c. Total operating revenue minus bad debts, charity, and contractual adjustments

   d. Gross operating revenues minus all deductions plus other operating revenues   _____

43. Productivity is computed by dividing full-time equivalent (FTE) employees (paid hours divided by 2,080) by the average daily census. A community hospital operating at a satisfactory level of productivity has

   a. 1–3 FTEs per occupied bed
   b. 2–3 FTEs per occupied bed
   c. 3–4 FTEs per occupied bed
   d. 4–5 FTEs per occupied bed   _____

44. The amount of debt that can usually be carried by a hospital is obtained by taking the annual principal and interest requirement divided by the total operating revenues. The guideline typically applied is

   a. 1–3 percent
   b. 3–5 percent
   c. 6–9 percent
   d. 10–12 percent   _____

45. Of the total community hospital beds in this country, the investor-owned health care corporations operate

   a. Approximately 10 percent
   b. Approximately 25 percent
   c. Approximately 40 percent
   d. Approximately 50 percent   _____

46. When annual capital budgets are prepared for the purchase of clinical equipment, physician participation is

   a. Not necessary
   b. Required by state medical practice acts
   c. A sound management philosophy
   d. Required by the governing authority   _____

47. The inpatient utilization rate of the age 65 and over cohort is

   a. Between 4,000 and 5,000 patient days per 1,000 persons

Answer

    b. Between 3,000 and 4,000 patient days per 1,000 persons

    c. Between 2,000 and 3,000 patient days per 1,000 persons

    d. Between 1,000 and 2,000 patient days per 1,000 persons   _____

48. On a national basis, Medicare patients typically account for what percentage of all patient days of care?

    a. 20–29 percent

    b. 30–39 percent

    c. 40–49 percent

    d. 50+ percent   _____

49. The percentage of inpatient admissions typically coming through a hospital emergency room is

    a. Less than 5 percent

    b. 6–10 percent

    c. 11–20 percent

    d. More than 20 percent   _____

50. Revenues from outpatient services, as a percentage of total operating revenue, typically are

    a. 1–8 percent

    b. 9–16 percent

    c. 17–25 percent

    d. More than 25 percent   _____

Number correct _____   Number incorrect _____

$\times \underline{2}$ _____

_____ %

I am a (check all that apply)

governing board member _____
physician   _____
member of management _____

Hospital Query Quotient Answer Key

Legal
1. a
2. d
3. b
4. c
5. a

Medical staff organization
6. c
7. c
8. c
9. b
10. d
11. d
12. b
13. b
14. d
15. c
16. a
17. c
18. b

19. a
20. c
21. c
22. b
23. c
24. d

Governing board organization
25. c
26. c
27. b
28. c
29. d
30. c
31. b
32. a

Patient care
33. d
34. c
35. a

36. a
37. b
38. c

General and financial
39. b
40. d
41. d
42. d
43. d
44. c
45. a
46. c
47. a
48. c
49. d
50. d

Index

Accreditation, 9, 81
Administrators. *See* Chief
  executive officers and
  administrators

Billing, 12–13

Chief executive officers and
  administrators, 5–6, 17, 19–
  20, 28–32, 35–36, 41–42, 47–
  49, 51–59, 61, 90–91, 109,
  11–12, 121, 133–35, 138–39,
  165–66, 167–68, 172, 183–84;
  medical staff and, 5, 9, 30–
  31, 47, 52, 56–58, 111, 116,
  139, 175–78, 182–83. *See also*
  Governing boards: chief
  executive officers and
  administrators and
Competition, 3–5, 15–23, 32–
  34, 36, 42–44, 46, 51, 56–57,
  62–63, 66, 69, 71, 76, 87,
  92–93, 97–100, 104, 106–7,
  122–23, 131, 147, 158, 184

Finances, 3–4, 6–7, 10–11,
  20–21, 23–35, 41, 43, 46, 48,
56–57, 59, 61–80, 82–83,
  92–93, 97–98, 100–102, 104,
  107, 109, 122–23, 128–29,
  132–33, 139, 141, 144–46,
  148–50, 153, 158, 166, 171,
  173, 179, 183–86; cost
  containment, 4, 8–9, 13; cost
  shifting, 6, 62, 82, 107, 148;
  discounting, 6, 10, 41, 44–
  45, 47, 51, 73, 145

Governing boards: chairperson, 45, 49, 51–59, 91, 106,
  108, 116, 122, 125, 132, 139,
  167–68, 180–81; chief
  executive officers and
  administrators and, 21–22,
  44–45, 47–49, 52–59, 105–8,
  110, 122, 125–27, 129, 134,
  139, 168, 180; committees,
  46–48, 52, 57, 102, 105–7,
  133, 179; compensation of
  members, 26, 102, 121, 128–
  31, 166, 181; composition,
  22, 42, 44–45, 47, 87–88, 92–
  93, 103, 105, 108; effectiveness, 35, 88–89, 91–94, 112,

About the Authors

Everett A. Johnson, Ph.D., FACHE, is the director of the Institute of Health Administration at the Georgia State University College of Business Administration. He is also director of The E.J. Group, Inc., a hospital and health care consulting firm in Marietta, Georgia. Before joining the Georgia State faculty, he was the chief executive officer of the Methodist Hospital in Gary, Indiana.

Everett Johnson has served as chairman of the board of governors of the American College of Healthcare Executives and as chairman of the board of trustees of the Indiana Hospital Association. His service to the field was recognized by the American College of Healthcare Executives in 1989 when he received the College's Silver Medal Award.

Richard L. Johnson, FACHE, is the president of TriBrook Group, Inc., a Chicago-based health care management consulting firm that he cofounded in 1972. In addition to 30 years as a health care consultant, his career has included the management of two major teaching institutions, the University of Chicago Hospitals, and the University of Missouri School of Medicine. He has served as an assistant director of the American Hospital Association and, during the Reagan administration, as health advisor to the secretary of the U.S. Air Force.

In 1983 Richard Johnson received the Silver Medal Award from the American College of Healthcare Executives, and in 1990 he was awarded the Award of Merit from the American Association of Healthcare Consultants. He has published five books and more than 100 articles based on his experiences.